WE
ARE
HAVING
THIS
CONVERSATION
NOW

THE TIMES
OF AIDS
CULTURAL
PRODUCTION

DUKE UNIVERSITY PRESS
DURHAM + LONDON 2022

WE
ARE
HAVING
THIS
CONVERSATION
NOW

ALEXANDRA
JUHASZ +
THEODORE
KERR

© 2022 Duke University Press
All rights reserved
Printed in the United States of America
on acid-free paper ∞
Designed by Aimee C. Harrison
Project editor: Annie Lubinsky
Typeset in Portrait Text Regular and
Folio Std by Copperline Book Services

Library of Congress Cataloging-in-Publication Data
Names: Juhasz, Alexandra, author. | Kerr, Theodore,
author.
Title: We are having this conversation now :
the times of AIDS cultural production /
Alexandra Juhasz and Theodore Kerr.
Description: Durham : Duke University Press,
2022. | Includes index.
Identifiers: LCCN 2021050864 (print) |
LCCN 2021050865 (ebook)
ISBN 9781478015840 (hardcover)
ISBN 9781478018483 (paperback)
ISBN 9781478023081 (ebook)
Subjects: LCSH: AIDS (Disease) in mass media. |
AIDS (Disease)—Social aspects—United States. |
AIDS (Disease)—Political aspects—United
States. | AIDS (Disease)—United States—
Historiography. | Health services accessibility—
Political aspects—United States. | AIDS
activists—United States. | BISAC: SOCIAL
SCIENCE / LGBTQ Studies / General |
PERFORMING ARTS / Film / History & Criticism
Classification: LCC P96.A39 J85 2022 (print) |
LCC P96.A39 (ebook) |
DDC 362.19697/92—dc23/eng/20220423
LC record available at
https://lccn.loc.gov/2021050864
LC ebook record available at
https://lccn.loc.gov/2021050865

Cover art: Chloe Dzubilo, *Calendar*.
Courtesy of the Fales Library and Special
Collections/Chloe Faith Dzubilo Papers
and the Estate of Chloe Dzubilo.

CONTENTS

ABBREVIATIONS

ACE	AIDS Counseling and Education Program
AE	Against Equality
AIDS	acquired immunodeficiency syndrome
APLA	AIDS Project Los Angeles
ASO	AIDS Service Organization
AZT	zidovudine, HIV antiviral medication
CAB	Client Advisory Board
CDC	Centers for Disease Control and Prevention
GMHC	Gay Men's Health Crisis
HAART	highly active antiretroviral therapy
HIM	Health Initiative for Men
HIV	human immunodeficiency virus
HRC	Human Rights Campaign
MSM	men who have sex with men
PAC	Prevention Access Campaign
PEPFAR	President's Emergency Plan for AIDS Relief
PREP	pre-exposure prophylaxis medication
PWA	People with AIDS
UNAIDS	Joint United Nations Programme on HIV/AIDS
VA	Visual AIDS
WAVE	Women's AIDS Video Enterprise

ACKNOWLEDGMENTS

This book is a conversation between us, Alex and Ted, as well as being a conversation with everyone we have had the pleasure of interacting with in our AIDS work along the way, and still others who we will meet on these pages. Please see our "Sources and Influences: Timeline 3" at the book's end to witness our creative attempt to situate ourselves in community and time, an ongoing preoccupation of this book, because it is so central to what we study, and how we do it, as feminist AIDS workers. If your name or work appears there or elsewhere in the book—in our conversations, footnotes, or prompts at each chapter's conclusion—know that this is only one small gesture of thanks for your sustaining contributions as writers, artists, thinkers, and activists. You make the world, and we think, our book, better. If your name is not here, this is not for want of needing you. Our community's work in AIDS cultural production is vast, over places and decades, and try as we could, we weren't able to find all the memories and citations we know are true to this sustaining output. The power of loss, and sometimes careful salvage, is central to this effort. Know that we know and thank you, even if we didn't name or find you.

In terms of foundational conversations, thank you to Elizabeth Ault at Duke University Press for your intelligent shepherding, and patience. Your encouragement and care over several years and many interactions have been so valuable to us. Thank you as well to all of our Duke readers. Your feedback helped to shape this book into what it is today. An earlier (and entirely different) iteration was also read at the University of Michigan Press. Thanks to Mary Francis for her interest in and support of our writing. We rewrote the book entirely after our first pass with the two presses, and while this was hard, we couldn't have gotten to what we have here without the difficult and encouraging feedback we received from peers.

This book comes out of seven years of writing together. Thank you to the editors and publishers who worked with us over the years as our ideas and processes concerning the Times of AIDS were taking shape, changing, and refining, including Gary Crowdus at *Cineaste*; Peter Knegt, formerly at Indie-

Wire; Jordan Lord at the Center for the Humanities, the Graduate Center, City University of New York (CUNY); Jennifer Patterson, Brighde Moffat, and Rachel Economy from Hematopoiesis Press; Angela Jones, who along with Joseph Nicholas DeFilippis and Michael W. Yarbrough worked with us on our essay for their three-part book series, *The Unfinished Queer Agenda after Marriage Equality*; Christopher Robé and Stephen Charbonneau, editors of *InsUrgent Media from the Front*; Poppy Coles, Mario Ontiveros, and Ellen Birrell at *X-Tra*; Cait McKinney and Marika Cifor for their issue of *First Mondays*; Nishant Shahani and Jih-Fei Cheng for including us in the dispatches on COVID-19 for the Duke University Press blog; and Bárbara Rodríguez Muñoz, editor of *Health* for Whitechapel: Documents of Contemporary Art.

We are so grateful to Lisa Cohen for reading an early draft of the book. Your sharp eye, honest feedback, and encouragement let us know that we should keep going. Thank you to Gavin McCormick for your care and attention as our last reader and copyeditor. Thank you also to Nava Renak for the refuge during our stay-at-home "retreat" in Ditmas Park, Brooklyn. We finished a version of the book in your home during COVID-19. We are also grateful to the various homeowners and retreat workers where we visited to write in seclusion and intensity over the years: in Hudson, Narrowsburg, and Phoenicia, New York; St. Louis, Missouri; and Pendle Hill in suburban Philadelphia. This time and your place was a gift we are grateful for. Our final "writing retreats" were held during COVID-19 over Zoom, and finally in our shared borough of Brooklyn.

Thank you to the organizers of the 2015 Media Fields conference at the University of California San Diego, where we first had the opportunity to share our ideas in front of a live audience, allowing us to get to begin to know each other in person on the train rides to and from LA, as well as over a memorable sunset beach walk. Similarly, we are grateful to the organizers of the 2016 conference After Marriage: The Future of LGBTQ Politics and Scholarship for the Center for LGBTQ Studies (CLAGS) at the City University of New York. Here we enjoyed an opportunity to engage our ideas about early activist AIDS video with an invested and generous audience eager to learn more. And while we did not present together, we also want to acknowledge Adam Geary, who along with Kristen Nelson put together the Dis-Orienting AIDS Discourse Symposium, hosted at the University of Arizona in 2015; and we want to thank our fellow presenters, Che Gossett, Eva Hayward, and Naina Khanna.

We owe a debt of gratitude to Visual AIDS and the extended community that the organization creates and cultivates, including T De Long who allowed us to use Chloe Dzubilo's work on the book cover. We are also grateful

x

to Caitlyn McCarthy at The Lesbian, Gay, Bisexual and Transgender Community Center, and Jennifer Gregg and Umi Hsu at the ONE Archives Foundation. Their support of our work—beginning with the *Metanoia* exhibition— helped provide us with the materials, time, walls, and processes from which to write our last chapter. We are also indebted to the many AIDS communities we thrive within, including Katherine Cheairs and Jawanza Williams, our co-curators on Metanoia, as well as the expansive world of What Would an HIV Doula Do? collective.

Alex gives thanks to: Brooklyn College, CUNY, and Pitzer College, for research funding that supported several of our writing retreats and travel to present our work. My family, colleagues, and friends for how you constitute the world in which I can think, connect, and stay safe. And Ted. When you interviewed me for an oral history on AIDS art, you helped me to express how James Robert (Jim) Lamb was my "best enabler." It turns out that I need and am lucky enough to receive more than one bearer of encouragement and life force over the changing Times of AIDS. For this, your enabling of my life in AIDS, I thank you.

Ted gives thanks to: Everyone who cares about, lives with, and works on HIV/AIDS. The people I have had the chance to work, organize, write, think, feel, and teach with. And of course, my friends and family for being interesting, and interested. Alex: We are older now than when we started. For that, I am grateful.

Alexandra Juhasz and Theodore Kerr have enjoyed a developing history of writing together. Many of the ideas shared in this book have their origins in the following coauthored works.

"I Made My Mourning Productive, Collective, and Interactive through Video Production . . . ," Visual AIDS (blog), February 5, 2013, https://visualaids.org/blog/i-made-my-mourning-productive -collective-and-interactive-through-video-prod.

"When ACT UP Is Remembered, Other Places, People, and Forms of AIDS Activism Are Disremembered: Part Two of an Interview with Queer Archive Activist Alexandra Juhasz," *Visual AIDS* (blog), February 17, 2013, https://www.thebody.com/article/when-act-up -is-remembered-other-places-people-and-.

"Home Video Returns: Media Ecologies of the Past of HIV/AIDS," *Cineaste* 39, no. 3 (2014), https://www.cineaste.com/summer 2014/home-video-returns-media-ecologies-of-the-past-of-hiv-aids.

"AIDS Reruns: Becoming 'Normal'? A Conversation on 'The Normal Heart' and the Media Ecology of HIV/AIDS," IndieWire, August 18, 2014, https://www.indiewire.com/2014/08/aids-reruns-becoming-normal-a-conversation-on-the-normal-heart-and-the-media-ecology-of-hivaids-216116/.

"Stacked on Her Office Shelf: Stewardship and AIDS Archives," Center for the Humanities, the Graduate Center, CUNY, January 13, 2017, https://www.centerforthehumanities.org/distributaries/stacked-on-her-office-shelf-stewardship-and-aids-archives.

"Who Are the Stewards of the AIDS Archives: Sharing the Political Weight of the Intimate," in *The Unfinished Queer Agenda: After Marriage Equality*, ed. Angela Jones, Joseph Nicholas DeFilippis, and Michael W. Yarbrough (London: Routledge, 2018), 88–101.

"Seeing What the Patrimony Didn't Save: Alternative Stewardship of the Activist Media Archive," in *InsUrgent Media from the Front*, ed. Chris Robé and Stephen Charbonneau (Bloomington: Indiana University Press, 2020), 87–105.

"On Care, Activism, and HIV," in *Health*, ed. Bárbara Rodríguez Muñoz (Cambridge, MA: MIT Press, 2020), 37–41.

"AIDS Normalization," *X-TRA* 22, no. 4 (Summer 2020), https://www.x-traonline.org/article/aids-normalization.

"Silence Doesn't Rhyme, but It Repeats: AIDS, BLM, COVID-19, and the Sound of What Is Missing, a Conversation in 4 Parts," Duke University Press blog, August 6, 2020, https://dukeupress.wordpress.com/2020/08/06/dispatches-on-aids-and-covid-19-continuing-conversations-from-aids-and-the-distribution-of-crises-dispatch-three/.

"Watching and Talking about AIDS: Analog Tapes, Digital Cultures, and Strategies for Connection," *First Monday* 25, no. 10 (October 5, 2020), https://doi.org/10.5210/fm.v25i10.10283.

THE TIMES
OF AIDS
TIMELINE 1

PRE-1981
AIDS BEFORE AIDS

The virus has been circulating within humans from as early as the 1900s in Cameroon, and as early as the late 1960s in the United States. There are lived experiences of HIV well before 1981, but these occur outside of discourse. Even so, a then-unnamed illness impacts individuals and communities.

1981–1987
THE FIRST SILENCE

In the early 1980s, medical staff and impacted people begin to take action around a mysterious health concern. Their work is done primarily in isolation. In the United States, co-ordinated efforts are blocked by the Reagan administration and an apathetic and uninformed media and public. The result: a once possibly manageable health crisis becomes an epidemic.

1987–1996
AIDS CRISIS CULTURE

From the "Silence = Death" poster to community-produced video and historic levels of direct action, this is a period of mass cultural production and discourse about HIV/AIDS leading to social, political, and medical breakthroughs.

1996–2008

THE SECOND SILENCE

The introduction of HAART (highly active antiretroviral therapy) produces better health for many and an associated decline in the space taken up by HIV in public. While HIV-related activity is ongoing it becomes, again, less connected and less visible.

2008–PRESENT

AIDS CRISIS REVISITATION

A sudden deluge of cultural production focused on earlier responses to the virus breaks the silence. Cultural production returns to the stories, images, and loss of the first generations. This is met with more excitement, criticism, connection. A richer understanding of AIDS—whether that be in terms of race, gender, sexuality, prevention, or undetectability—enters discourse.

2016–PRESENT

AIDS [CRISIS] NORMALIZATION

Mentions of AIDS become more commonplace, expected, and present-invested within US culture. The HIV response takes on a more stable and integrated place in discourse. AIDS is less connected to trauma. It is understood as one problem among many. It is placed into history. AIDS as crisis is present but less definitive, even as stigma, discrimination, and criminalization organize the lives of some people living with HIV.

Time is not a line. We offer this timeline to be helpful, not prescriptive. AIDS is not over.

INTRODUCTION
WE ARE STARTING THIS CONVERSATION, AGAIN

This is a book about the history, present, and future of the cultural production of AIDS. It takes the form of thirteen short conversations between two AIDS activists, Alex and Ted, whom you will get to know more as you go along. The book focuses on what we call the Times of AIDS. All this talk is inspired by our longtime AIDS activism and is initiated by looking at related cultural production: objects like AIDS activist videos; events like protests; spaces like AIDS memorials; ideas we have learned from within and outside our community; and through our own memories and hopes. Our book relies on conversation as a method that helps us better understand AIDS, ourselves, others, history, and more; this, so we can work together to help improve the lives of people living with HIV/AIDS and respect the memory of those who have died and struggled. It is a book that invites you to join in this conversation, art, and action. Each short chapter ends with a prompt or a set of questions, as well as some resources that might inspire you to question and also engage. But before all that, we begin our conversation with three opening questions that we will also answer. We want to create an opportunity for readers and writers alike to situate themselves as we start in a shared and participatory interaction with this book. For your part, answer some, many, or none of these and further prompts; answer them before you begin; or return (again) when you are ready.

1 Why did you pick up this book? What do you bring to it?
2 How and with whom do you talk about AIDS?
3 What do you think are methods or practices that allow for progressive social change?

WHY DID YOU PICK UP THIS BOOK?
WHAT DO YOU BRING TO IT?

We wrote this book because both of us—activist mediamaker and scholar Alexandra Juhasz and writer and organizer Theodore Kerr—have committed our lives to the AIDS epidemic and the people, communities, and culture that have been changed through it. We do this as two white, formally educated, middle- and upper-middle-class queer, HIV-negative people of different cis genders and generations. Over decades, we have each brought our lived perspectives to diverse communities where we work to name, negotiate, and account for our differences from and similarities with our AIDS colleagues, often through conversation, art, or action. We work in diverse communities to change the impacts of AIDS among us. Our whiteness, our negative sero status, our sexualities, as well as our cities and educations, give us specific but adaptable perspectives and privileges that we share in our work, and also here. We also bring our ideological perspectives to our AIDS work. We share commitments to eradicating anti-Black racism and furthering queer analysis. This means our work is grounded in intersectional feminism, taking our cues from the 1977 Combahee River Collective statement and its lineage of thinkers, artists, and activists:[1] "The most general statement of our politics at the present time would be that we are actively committed to struggling against racial, sexual, heterosexual, and class oppression, and see as our particular task the development of integrated analysis and practice based upon the fact that the major systems of oppression are interlocking." To this analysis we add HIV, and our own experiences, since we are at once quite different from each other, just as we are aligned through beliefs, values, and aspirations for a world where the harm of HIV is eradicated. As people with different bodies, experiences, ideas, communities, and commitments, we have been changed in context and time. Much of this transformation has come through our engagements with AIDS culture, specifically, objects that allow for conversation about HIV. To our book we bring and try to model this history, and our commitment to these processes. We want to share this with you in your own specific and adaptable situation vis-à-vis AIDS.

HOW AND WITH WHOM DO YOU TALK ABOUT AIDS?

We talk about AIDS as writers, educators, mediamakers, activists, and friends. We talk over the phone, via texts, emails, and video chat. Sometimes we talk together in person. We are always also engaging with others. Primarily, though, this book shows how we talk together about AIDS through and as our work, which began in an online conversation in 2013.[2] We have continued to do this ever since, through ten published essays, multiple public events, in activist collectives, and of course, here and now. As individuals, Alex, an activist, scholar, and videomaker, has been focused for decades on the concerns raised by women and AIDS. This has meant that her work has been grounded in intersectional feminism, the development of queer studies and activism, her connections to communities of color, and a commitment to a media praxis. Ted, a writer and organizer, found and formed his bearings working first at an AIDS service organization in Canada that was rooted in the understanding—and practice—that AIDS is an intersectional issue that includes sexuality, race, and gender, as well as poverty and class.

We look at and contribute to AIDS cultural production: work that takes place primarily outside the realms of science and government (although it may speak to these institutions). This means we are invested in the harder-to-quantify labor and output of artists, activists, care workers, archivists, and thinkers. Taking place in the fields of arts, humanities, health, and advocacy, we meet in our "AIDS work," a phrase we borrow from historian Jennifer Brier to refer to the labor performed by people "expressly committed to addressing the effects of AIDS."[3]

WHAT DO YOU THINK ARE METHODS OR PRACTICES THAT ALLOW FOR PROGRESSIVE SOCIAL CHANGE?

We have found that exploring AIDS through time and conversation creates the conditions we need to contribute to progressive social change. "The Times of AIDS: Timeline 1" opens the book. We developed this as a framework to explore experiences with cultural production about the epidemic; we developed this as we were making sense of decades of diverse AIDS cultural production that varied in process, audience, and goals.

We used conversation as an invitation to listen, learn, and share, and as an activity that can engender surprise, change, learning, emotion, and yes, sometimes being annoyed or triggered. Along the way we have learned that

3

conversation can be an argument or a love fest, a place to be wrong or to learn more, an engagement in which feelings are hurt or repaired. A conversation can be clarifying or confusing, and when you are lucky, it can stay with you for a long time or open you into new understandings unreachable without it.

Conversation is a process.

As curious and social people, conversation has been a tool acquired over years. We have cultivated it through informal and social means, as well as professionally through teaching, and through our activism, which is collaborative, iterative, and engaged. We have honed conversation through friendship; love affairs; work experiences; by living in various cities; engaging with a diversity of technologies; through our work as students and educators; in exchanges where we have led and shared ideas and those where we follow and listen; and through years of shared work together and in this particular writing format.

Conversation rooted to social change is what we practice and also hope to engender.

It is through conversation that we were able to move across time together and within our broader communities. For of course, the making of this book—and our work toward progressive social change—was never limited to conversation between just us. In writing this book we had conversations with friends, artists, AIDS service organization employees, and activists, as well as editors, other academics, writers, and the many anonymous readers who helped us better understand this book. We've conversed with cultural artefacts from all the Times of AIDS. And we extend the possibility of conversation to you as a reader. As we have mentioned, at the end of every chapter (and at the beginning of this one as well!), even as the book moves forward linearly, we ask you to stop, and talk. To review, search, consider, relate, and record. We offer questions and resources to trigger (more on this term, its histories, multiple meanings, and associated affects soon) your participation. Your conversation will have its own revelations, hiccups, places of vulnerability or impasse; you might want, find, and use different words that help you to best engage with these ideas or with another person; you might argue with or expand upon what we lay out here, starting below with our Times of AIDS.

Do you want to have this conversation now?

THE TIMES AND TIMELINES OF AIDS

4   It was through conversation that we came to appreciate the fundamental role of time in understanding and using AIDS cultural production. That led us to craft, refine, and share our Times of AIDS. This is a chronological framework

for understanding what HIV has been, is now, and what we strive for it to become. "The Times of AIDS: Timeline 1" is one of three timelines we share in this book, and for us it is a crystallization of our thinking. This is why it opens our book. We will develop, embellish, challenge, and open out this compact formation across the thirteen conversations that follow. We will ask you to do the same. To begin, flip back a few pages to familiarize yourself with the timeline, knowing that your questions, places of connection, and possible discomfort and critique are critical.

Delineating AIDS cultural production in this way helps us to learn from what can otherwise be experienced as a vast, confusing, and overwhelming body of work that exists in the past and present. In the conversations that follow, we periodize from our own felt experiences of and in time as we encounter each other and traces of the past. We also use larger medical, political, and cultural breakthroughs as markers. Then again, many small moments or pieces of art stimulate our consideration. We use each encounter, to place it and ourselves in time. Feeling our engagement, learning with objects, relaying this encounter with precision and detail: all this has helped us to see and settle ourselves, our experiences, and our AIDS work, in time(s).

We propose the Times of AIDS less as tight periods than as fruitful processes, less as benchmarks and more as ways to understand how AIDS can be experienced and has changed over its decades-long history, and whenever you encounter it in the present. Informing our thinking around the creation of this timeline (and two more that follow), and so also the book, is the idea that time is not a line.[4] Yes, sometimes it moves through our world and bodies with a steady forward beat. And time is certainly known and felt linearly: we age, things change, nothing lasts. However, time can also be felt, known, and used in creative, collaborative, and flexible ways that we also find descriptive and productive. It can be saved in things or people for others to learn from, and use again. We can revisit and make good use of earlier times that have been stored in our records, our art, our bodies. Time can hold us together, in our difficult but always glorious present and across our many differences, so that we can better know each other and the world. It provides the horizon for action and change.

We have been challenged with love by friends, readers, and peers about our urge to periodize. We take these comments seriously. We agree that time cannot be standardized. The Times of AIDS are porous, loose, interdependent, co-constitutive. But when hard work is needed to create a better future, it can be useful to make sense of the present by taking stock of the past: accounting for patterns, forces, events, and anomalies that indicate how both

5

power and people affect things, ourselves, and others. We think the Times of AIDS serve as one useful lens to better see AIDS, as well as other viruses, crises, or movements. For of course HIV/AIDS has deep, lasting, and complex connections with other traumas, pandemics, health inequities, and blights of systemic inequality. And just as AIDS links to other issues, we think all of the periods of AIDS are themselves linked, ongoing, and co-present. That is: Silence remains with us across all these Times; Revisitation can be fruitful for understanding the impact of viruses in the present; AIDS Crisis Culture, while occurring over a relatively short period, has had a long impact.

Once we had committed to our first timeline we found that we needed to get creative to represent how that effort only partially answered the questions about time that motivated our conversations. We needed other formats that could be responsive to how time felt in our ongoing and changing AIDS work, and how we make use of objects from all the Times of AIDS, mixed together, or regardless of "order," to better understand and change the pandemic. So you will encounter two more timelines, each quite different in style and scope.

"An AIDS Conversation Script to Be Read Aloud: Timeline 2" takes the form of a dialogue. Holding its place in the middle of the book, it also serves as a break, a challenge, a transition. Unlike the other two, this timeline is not linear; it is presentational. It is also one of many pauses for reflection and interaction that we offer as routes to conversation about AIDS. Given its format, we hope that you might not just read but also perform the timeline with another or others before you progress back into the more linear Time(s) of the book. "Sources and Influences: Timeline 3" is our last act. It is a creative rendering of something like a bibliography and mediography. A representative but not exhaustive list of many of the cultural influences that taught, moved, or changed us or our AIDS worlds (books, texts, video, film, exhibitions, and what we call "projects," which include events, groups, meetings, websites, and more), ordered by year, it strives to demonstrate the situatedness of our own and others' AIDS work in time, culture, and community. Thinking and writing alongside related works of scholarly/activist practice and publication, for instance Katherine McKittrick's "Footnotes (Books and Papers Scattered About the Floor)," our third timeline, and other creative practices of citation we have chosen to use in the book, "when understood as *in conversation* with each other, demonstrate an interconnected story that resists oppression."[5]

Our three timelines gesture at how our book is both metaphysical and practical: How do you represent time; how can time be useful for social change; how can you think in and about time with others; how can this

6

thinking, writing, remembering, and engaging with culture in community help change AIDS?

TRIGGER AND SILENCE

The book comprises two parts, "Trigger" and "Silence," that move linearly through our Times of AIDS. "Trigger" focuses on AIDS Crisis Culture, as well as what preceded it, the First Silence. "Silence" links the Second Silence with AIDS Crisis Revisitation, anticipating and bringing us to AIDS [Crisis] Normalization. By moving forward using the Western calendar, we take up one metric to display the pulse of AIDS cultural production that we felt and still feel, with a particular focus on our own experiences of noticeable or missing work, neglect, pause, and quiet, as well as of action, voice, and connection. Moving together in this way through our experiences—from voice, to silence, to voice again; from connection, to isolation, to new movements and visibility—revealed a critical insight: the dominant role played by silence throughout AIDS history. Look above; silence is always with us when it comes to AIDS.

In Part One, "Trigger," our close, careful work is with one videotape, title unknown, made around 1990 by a community-based AIDS organization in Philadelphia first known as BEBASHI, Blacks Educating Blacks about Sexual Health Issues (now known as Bebashi: Transition to Hope). This videotape guides our considerations of the vast output of AIDS Crisis Culture and more importantly our process with objects from the past via conversation, the ethical ways we try to engage with the bountiful production from this and every period. We let the tape lead us; we trust its knowledge; we learn from its recorded present, as well as from the many absences that the uncredited and unnamed makers of the tape have left behind.

Engaging with the tape as it engaged with its subject matter, actors, and audience, we became interested in the afterlife of an object, which for us means: considering the makers of the tape; how the tape depicts caregivers and caregiving, representation and representing; and the respectful regard we provide the tape as a method of research and engagement. Over its six chapters we model different practices of considered attention and mediated conversation that we learn from and use for the AIDS work we do here. Throughout these interactions with each other and the tape, we consider how videotapes itself is a tool engendering a variety of practices for historical, personal, and community attention across the cultural production of AIDS.

7

Part One is primarily concerned with video, the ways it serves as both object and process to help save and generate social change for people living with AIDS and their communities. We understand AIDS activist videotapes, and the processes that make, save, find, and share them, across time and AIDS communities, as political, tactical, and ethical. We engage together, guided by the many ways the tape models conversation for its viewers, including speaking with another or others with generosity, vulnerability, negotiation, and attention. Importantly, and perhaps counterintuitively, this tape is pretty brutal. We see Black women in Philadelphia navigating the realities of getting sick and dying from AIDS while struggling with poverty, racism, sexism, and domestic and systemic violence. It doesn't model care for its viewers in ways more common in our cultural production today. Rather, it shows suffering, it renders violence, it produces agitation, and there is little to no catharsis.

To engage with its hard ideas and its careful approach to them, we turn to rich traditions of thought and activism including archival and memorial studies, feminist intersectionality, histories and theories of videotape, the PWA (People with AIDS) empowerment movement, and a rich body of scholarly and community-based work about HIV/AIDS across a range of disciplines. A media ecology perspective allows us the space to engage with well-known art from this era, even as we spend time with lesser-known works whose impact can be reclaimed and circulated again. Learning with the tape, we model vulnerability as subject and method. We place ourselves, as white viewers, in relationship to this tape about and by Black women and their communities. In looking at and striving to account for the ongoing and changing effects of identity, we embrace our commitment to name how anti-Blackness and white supremacy—along with misogyny, homophobia, and other biases—affect the health, wealth, and representation of people living with and impacted by HIV. This also requires us to bring in and converse with our peers. Outside of the considered reading and watching we have already mentioned, we chose to contact and engage with present-day employees of Bebashi. Because one of our interviewees opens out new connections and memories, we end with more questions. We learn to honor absence, to see it as information. These foci on loss, memorial, and identity result in conversations around who gets seen, remembered, and ignored—and for the good of the living or the dead? We briefly share the story of Katrina Haslip, a Black woman living with HIV who, working from Bedford prison with others on the inside and outside, helped expand the definition of AIDS so that by 1993, more women and other people with HIV could access the resources and recognition they needed to live, thrive, and die with dignity. Haslip will return again, at the close of Part Two, a central player in our show *Metanoia*. We memorialize as we go; our linear work loops.

To put the Bebashi tape into context and conversation with its time, we connect it to more than fifty contemporaneous media objects from AIDS Crisis Culture: videos, newsletters, posters, and educational campaigns. In this way we explore what is extraordinary (and ordinary) about this one tape. But the Bebashi video, it turned out, served us all on its own, and as we most needed. The uncredited makers of this tape did their AIDS work using methods and formats that we learn from and understand as useful for us today: peer-to-peer; honoring local knowledge and vernacular; dialogic; and mediated, recorded, and made and saved to be used. They recorded themselves in conversation to document their ideas and AIDS culture in Black Philadelphia in the 1980s so as to help themselves, as well as to create and share a legacy.

In the tape we encounter three vignettes, each ending in media res, opening a door for viewers to talk among themselves about what they just saw and what they—in that position—would, or perhaps will, do. The tape models a dialogical form of intimate and urgent engagement that we activate again now. In the parlance of the 1980s and 1990s, the Bebashi tape was understood as a "trigger tape," a practice of using media within a community-based interaction to instigate potentially life-saving conversations between impacted people. Three "triggers" in the tape—overt ruptures and opportunities to pause the action on the screen—were placed to initiate a process of audience engagement, led by a facilitator, where viewers could share their own reflections and knowledge about what they had just seen. This form proved to be inspirational for us and for our book. A trigger tape invites reckoning, conversation, and potential growth for its anticipated audience.

We carry forward the AIDS work of the Bebashi videomakers by mirroring this tactic. First, we do this ourselves, in our conversations, as we meet each other on the page. Ask questions. Stop. Consider. As we write taking up a conversational format, we aim to be neither didactic nor prescriptive. This is one of the strengths of conversation: it assumes that participants have things to say and share, much they know, and also much to learn. In this way, we illustrate that a process of learning is as important as its content. And as we've said, after this introduction, and then after each of our thirteen chapters, we end each with triggers for you. For some, trigger has been understood as an abrupt, powerful, but careful invitation to engage, emerge from silence or isolation, and talk with others about AIDS in community. Today a "trigger warning" provides people space and time to learn when and as they feel

9

ready. Care undergirds both tactics, as does trauma. AIDS was and still is a catastrophe, a crisis, a scourge. Being in its proximity, living with it, talking about it, is not easy, nor always pleasant, even as we will argue that it can be transformative. We understand that conversation about AIDS can be difficult, painful, intense. We demonstrate these feelings and hurdles in our thirteen conversations, and we acknowledge that these and other feelings will most likely be part of your experience of our writing, and the interactions you may have if you follow our prompts at each chapter's end.

Because of the difficult—if powerful and sometimes empowering—emotions, memories, and processes we are learning about, engaging in, and asking you to try as we talk about AIDS through the Bebashi tape, between Parts One and Two we offer a pause for reflection and also for engagement and interaction: a way to think and do differently with our book, a method for creativity, performance, and being together. "An AIDS Conversation Script to Be Read Aloud: Timeline 2" also serves as a conceptual bridge into and about the primary subject of Part Two, "Silence." Here we focus upon the next two intertwined Times of AIDS cultural production: the Second Silence + AIDS Crisis Revisitation. In its seven chapters we do not celebrate silence, even as we acknowledge its motivating power. We begin by speaking broadly, at times theoretically, at times antagonistically, about the nature of silence. We grapple to define silence. We are moved to the personal. We listen and argue. Silence is dark, destructive, and generates shame, guilt, and doubt, but sometimes also possibility. Our conversation helps us learn something we found very hard as writers and activists: naming silence is a contradiction in terms.

As we were writing the book, our arduous path to understanding silence often ended in failure. For the life of us, we couldn't find, let alone settle on one useful object to ground, focus, and build our conversation as we had in Part One. But in this absence, there was much to learn. First, we discovered our silences are different. Even as we are both AIDS activists, our experiences and memories of the Second Silence are private, unique, at times painful or shameful, and disconnected from the other's and others. We found that to exit silence's thrall we needed to speak, share, and learn from our own and then the other's silence. Because here is the thing about silence: it is not absence; it is not lack. Silence is full, powerful, and in this way wreaks havoc within all the Times of AIDS. Silence persists. Silence defines AIDS culture. These hard-won lessons grew into the second part of this book. Our method adapted, and we turned to and relied more on our personal experiences. Because this process was so hard, overwhelming, and painful, you will see that its writing, tone, and feeling differs from the first part.

Our book is built upon, within, and against the Second Silence, which is bracketed by periods of intense cultural production that came before and after it: AIDS Crisis Culture and the Revisitation. We struggled, by definition, to see silence. In the struggle we grew to understand that the Second Silence was a period of culturally and individually produced isolation and underproduction, but also, importantly, ongoing activity. In particular, the communities that have always been hardest hit by HIV/AIDS—women, people of color, trans people, people of the global South, sex workers—continued to do their AIDS work in this period. They were not silent; they were speaking, working, and representing because the AIDS crisis persisted and grew in this period of silence, a long period where support, attention, and possibilities for connection suddenly evaporated for everyone, but particularly for those with less access to funds, institutions, and medication. So even when work was produced in this challenging Time that followed a period of more abundance, it often flamed out, lacking response, community, oxygen.

The second half of Part Two was easier. We had at last arrived at the period and the questions that had first drawn us together: AIDS Crisis Revisitation. In the chapters that focus on this Time, we think about the significant body of cultural production that has come from and after silence. We focus on a few select cultural objects to do so, again choosing depth over breadth. In fact, we end by closely considering an art show that we co-curated, with Katherine Cheairs and Jawanza Williams, during the months when we were finishing a complete draft of the book. The last chapter attends to our archival art show *Metanoia: Transformation through AIDS Activism and Archives* (2019 in New York and 2020 in Los Angeles, with online and other publications and events still being generated and shared).[6] We detail how we tried to expand the conversation we'd been having between the two of us while writing this book to incorporate a larger, more diverse team of AIDS workers, as well as different practices of presentation that might be useful for a range of anticipated local and digital audiences. This work, like much that we value most, forefronts the voices and histories of those most impacted and least represented. Our show and our conversation about it here highlight the largely forgotten histories of Black female prison activists who advocated for their own healthcare and compassionate release during AIDS Crisis Culture, a time of abundant production (for some) in which silence was still theirs to break.

11

OBJECT AND CITATION

Cultural objects hold information, stories, and also legacies of power and pride, voice, and silence. They allow us to better understand who gets to speak and how and when are they heard. Who is remembered. Whose voice is lost. An object from the past—and its makers, subjects, anticipated users—perhaps neglected, is located, discussed, and witnessed with rigor, with honor, and in depth, in our best effort to move it carefully to our use, now, all the while respecting its unique history, authors, and context. We attempt to learn from, attend to, and better the abuses of power that live in all acts of culture—representation, preservation, history-making, theory-writing, conversation—acknowledging that there is always more to learn, always ways to improve, always more transparency, honesty, and communication to be had, and always differences in power and control depicted in objects and what we do with them. We seek processes and resources that help us to see, name, and counter the interlocked systems of oppression in which we, and the things we and others make and save, are situated. We model strategies for engaging with cultural objects from all the Times of AIDS through an interpersonal process rooted in intentionality and attentiveness,[7] time travel and deep witnessing. This method allows us, together and in conversation, to better see the epidemic in the present and the past through multiplying perspectives, including our own.

For instance, much of the current history of AIDS (and the Revisitation that writes it) has been animated by gay white men: their stories, resources, archival holdings, and contemporary needs. Our conversational model begins by noting our place in a history we both contribute to, celebrate, and criticize, as white, queer, HIV-negative activists. We then work to consider an object's place within legacies of ownership, theft, reclamation, revisitation, and ongoing self-determination for marginalized and affected people and communities. We believe that responsibility for any object is shared and never owned. Rather, when talking about a video, a moment in time, or an art show, we strive to free a thing from being someone's property or as being singular in itself; at the same time, working to respect a creator's and audiences' needs, intentions, and contexts. We know that most things people do and make to save themselves and others will be lost—as were many of these people—even as they struggled, persevered, and made powerful AIDS work, with and within beauty, anger, and community. Through conversation, what has been lost can be reclaimed, or at least revisited.

With this in mind, we also work with citation as another method to account for legacies of theft and control, as well as coming into and owning voice and connection. In her radical thinking about citation and activist intellectual method, McKittrick writes: "When we are doing our very best work, we are acknowledging the shared and collaborative intellectual praxis that makes our research what it is."[8] As is true for her creative scholarly method, we too have chosen to take up three complementary methods of citation to mark our thinking about and commitments to understanding cultural work politically. These idiosyncratic citation methods provide further information about the objects we discuss, while situating our writing in a broader AIDS community and history of cultural work. First: you will find that in our conversation we only occasionally cite sources. We have chosen to honor how and when we share inspiration vernacularly, when we are chatting informally with a friend or colleague. We include footnotes to our conversations when we actually refer to a specific publication or quotation. Second: at the end of each short chapter we offer you a few select readings, viewings, and associated activities. These point to work from our many peers that we think expands and enriches our discussion. Finally, our book ends with "Sources and Influences: Timeline 3." This is a modified bibliography and mediography of the AIDS cultural production that has informed and inspired us as writers and activists. Like Timeline 1, here we think chronologically about the work that has influenced this book.

We put more effort than you might otherwise know into formulating, refining, and naming our distinct methods to engage with objects and citation—methods that we believe honor and reflect our commitments to time, community, and AIDS cultural production. Like our timelines, we are sure our methods and formats will produce conversation, and most likely debate, within our communities. We invite and relish your engagement.

WE RETURN AND END WITH THE TIMES OF AIDS

As of winter 2021, there are 38 million people across the globe living with HIV; more than 74 million people have been diagnosed with HIV since records of this sort started to be kept. These large-scale numbers, built one by one from the loss and suffering of individuals and their communities, are a reminder that before HIV is an area of study, or a focus of culture, or a matter of conversation; it is a material, bodily reality. HIV lives in some people's bodies and not in others; in some communities in greater numbers than others;

13

and in some regions or places where it amplifies incredible stress upon already weakened systems. There are different costs and different experiences of any one diagnosis. Viruses are themselves rooted in formative systems of bias and deprivation dependent on race, gender, sexuality, geography, and much more.

As of now there is no cure for HIV, although there is a medical treatment developed decades into its history with its own costs and benefits. HAART can severely reduce the burden of the virus on a person's body. But AIDS is not over. Regardless of pills, cures, or vaccines, HIV disproportionately taxes some humans' daily lives due to systemic injustice, and is suffered disproportionately through stigma, discrimination, and criminalization. For these violations there is also no cure; only treatment, through culture.

We are not comfortable with popular public health and wellness campaign rhetoric that works toward goals like being "HIV free" or "ending AIDS." We are sensitive to what such terms mean for all the people who have ever lived with HIV. We know these terms discount the experiences of people currently living with the virus. They ignore people who will get a positive diagnosis in the future. However, we also understand and support the hope behind these words. One day, the crisis of AIDS will be over. In that Time of AIDS—No AIDS—there will be no more diagnoses, no more stigma. Suffering with HIV will end. The Times of AIDS will be over. At the Time of No AIDS, what we will have, what will remain as ours to keep, save, and share, will be the power, knowledge, art, and connection that we accrued across the waves of viral and linked crises encountered by our bodies, in our communities, in our cultural production, and in time. Others will be able to use this.

Until AIDS is over, acts and processes of attention, connection, healing, and empowerment that have been refined over the Times of this crisis can and should be used now. Our book tries to learn from, engage in, and model the best of such practices honed from our noble traditions, some of which we have named ourselves, and which we share with the hopes of propagating more. When AIDS is over, the book and all of those remarkable objects and processes will remain as a useful guide to how humans struggle to save themselves and each other. The Times of AIDS, and this conversation about it, are processes for interactive engagements with cultural artifacts from the past and present of AIDS aimed at saving ourselves and bettering our world. We invite you to join us in this conversation, now.

14

PARTICIPATE IN THE TIMES OF AIDS

We offer interactions with Timeline 1. This is our first of many such invitations to join the conversation, and thereby generate more interaction, knowledge, and possibility.

1 **REVIEW**
   "The Times of AIDS: Timeline 1"

2 **CONSIDER**
   Which of the six Times of AIDS resonates the most with how and when you came to understand the epidemic?

3 **SEARCH**
   A significant body of work about AIDS offers timelines as a way to understand the crisis. Find one or more "AIDS timelines" and consider what this rendering of history, memory, and culture makes visible.

4 **RELATE AND RECORD**
   As you engage with "The Times of AIDS: Timeline 1," consider doing the following:
   - keep a journal
   - call a friend and discuss
   - make art in response
   - use a format with which you are comfortable

We suggest relating and recording at each chapter's end as a way to further engage with our prompts.

PART
ONE
TRIGGER

TRIGGER 1
WHAT WE SEE

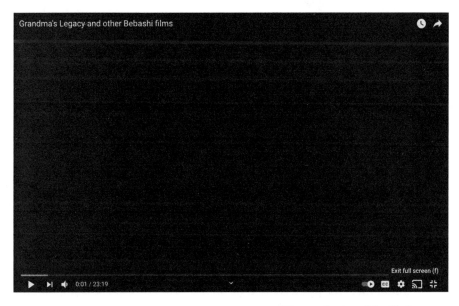

I.I The tape begins with a black screen.

THEODORE (TED) KERR **begins the conversation:** There is a blank screen. And silence. Then, an audible arrival of low static, the sound of space being recorded. Another switch in sound introduces a different pitch of static that will remain constant throughout the rest of the tape. A tall Black woman, with brown eyes and her hair pulled back, appears on the screen from a fade-up. We see her on the phone with her arm in a sling. A young girl in a solid-colored sweatshirt, the daughter we soon learn, plays with large blocks on the floor. The actors are surrounded by a set meant to convey home: a table with plates and cutlery, a couch, and a room divider. All is muted in VHS-grade blues, browns, and yellows. The tape's lack of crispness means that patterns on fabrics are slightly smudged. Everything is actually a little blurry and doesn't ever fully resolve into focus. Instead, as viewers, we adjust. We are invited into their video world and we choose to pay attention.

ALEXANDRA (ALEX) JUHASZ continues: We choose to stay for a number of reasons: this place and time and the video that holds it all feel authentic, a tad vulnerable, and thus long gone, a way of being on tape no longer possible because it isn't at all self-aware and has no aspirations for a significant viewership or even professionalism. Part of its pull also comes from the ways that nostalgia seems to adhere so definitively to anything on VHS tape. It had such a short life. Its visual and even aural textures are obvious, unique, and stuck in the 1980s, registering a very specific yesterday, with its brash but fading colors, its dirty pixelations, its smudges of data and kitschy confidence.

TED: VHS video was an aesthetic I was born into; it warms up my senses, providing me with a strong feeling of familiarity, a location in terms of time and space.

ALEX: Weird. Video feels so cold to me, dead as it must be. Sure, it connects me to a time I remember, but one that was hard and cruel when I was living it, and then also hard and cruel now but in a different way. As much as I might want, I have little access (beyond tapes) to this time which is also my young adulthood. These tapes, and the world they re-render, look really different from and dated in relation to today's video and world, and since I was there, I'm marked, too. And I certainly don't want to be nostalgified, which usually feels belittling or at least a little condescending. In this tape, the look of the video, the acting style of the actress, the inflection of her voice, confirm for me that it was something between educational and home video, a mode from the past of video that is often now either idealized or satirized or both. There was no hope that the tape would begin someone's YouTube career, or get loads of hits. It's crystal-clear that she's not exactly an actor even though she's performing.

TED: And it's not clear if there's a script or if they are improvising. "Girl, I'm about at the end of my rope," she proclaims dramatically into the phone. A wide shot follows where we see the child continuing to play. The mother holds the receiver close to her face with one hand and clutches the phone cord with the other. She is stuck in an abusive relationship and looking for a chance to vent—as well as another place to stay, just in case. She is determined. There is an audible disruption as static rumbles deeper for a beat. The woman reports that her husband is coming back home. She instructs her daughter to clean up her toys.

ALEX: Her man did not return home last night and this causes her distress not only because she does not know where he was but because of the disrespect his absence shows her in their relationship.

TED: She begins to scurry around making sure the house is clean. She becomes agitated. For the first time I notice the shadow of the actress moving against the back wall of the set. As a man enters, he walks across and through what seems to be the major light source.

ALEX: This is a noticeable hallmark of what I have, in my work on YouTube, called "bad video" (lovingly, don't get me wrong; Hito Steyerl's "defense of the poor image" is also critical here):[1] where the cheap seams of media production by nonprofessionals become glaringly obvious, and in so doing anchor to the tape or perhaps its viewing an authenticity but also a kind of triviality and expendability in today's oversaturated media culture. That would not be the case when it was first viewed. Then, we weren't overwhelmed by media representations. People would have been awed by the fact of their community's representation in and of itself: that poor and working-class Black women were on the screen, something hardly ever seen, at least without disdain and judgment.

TED: You are suggesting that when the tape was made people would not have noticed that the top of his shoulders and head are too brightly illuminated.

ALEX: Notice and not. The fact of it being an honest rendition of a known but largely unseen media narrative would prevail over aesthetic judgments. But even more so, his immediate, insisting dominance is what is most notable, I'd warrant, for any viewer.

TED: True, certainly for me. For the rest of the scene I see the hot glare of the unmoving white light where his body once absorbed the heat at the same time that I observe his power.

ALEX: He is a lumbering figure whose presence sticks everywhere. His face is that of a well-trained stoic masking a storm just below the surface. He's really scary. And where she initially stood firm, solid, and centered, his body and voice now dominate the room and she becomes unexpectedly and immediately small in the face of his withheld fury.

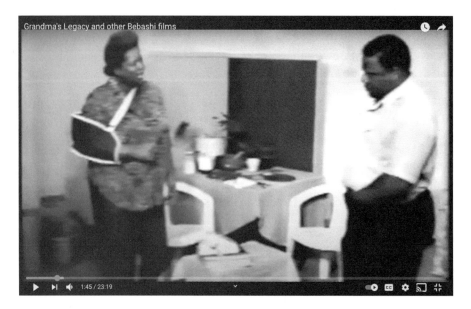

1:45 / 23:19

1.2 The first vignette takes an unflinching look at domestic violence.

TED: But his restraint is short-lived. He quickly becomes rough, accusing her of hiding a man in their house. Using what she has—her voice, words, and touch—she tries to defuse his anger. As the scene progresses, she gently asks where he was last night, to which he responds by verbally abusing her, reminding her that he already broke one arm and is willing to break the other.

ALEX: Our attention is no longer on the bad lighting. Things are raw emotionally and are driving forward in a very bad way. His anger turns toward the child. The woman puts herself between her daughter and the man, collecting the girl and taking her off-screen. When the mother returns, she again attempts to mollify him. This first scenario fades to black as she draws her man into a vivid, heated, clothed, but highly sexual embrace.

TED: From the earlier phone call, we know she has a place she could go if she needs to leave. But we don't know if she ever gets there. The scene ends before her story does.

ALEX: It's a dramatic, awful, dark, and honest start that ends on the same black screen with which the tape started.

TED: We are left not knowing what she will do, and put into a position where we might question our own choices if we were in her situation.

TRIGGER ONE

ALEX: But after this dip to black, the family, and all their myriad tensions, uncertainties, and realms of danger, vanish from the screen. We are introduced to a new actress: also African American, older and with short straight hair. She is sitting in front of what was the room divider in the previous scene, now serving as a wall. The sign behind her reads, "Shelter Rules." Again, the action starts on the phone, but this time the actress speaks centered in the frame and within one single long take, an impressive feat of acting and direction.

TED: She is speaking with Spike, a man with whom she too has a complicated and violent relationship. At first her tone is calm. She asks him to try to find her medical card. She needs it so she can get into a rehab facility. As the conversation continues it is clear she hopes to get the card with as little interaction with Spike as is possible. Meanwhile, he is using the card as ransom. He wants to see her again. She remains carefully upbeat. As the conversation sways between her current needs and their shared past, she thanks him repeatedly for treating her well when they were both using drugs. But she also reflects upon when things between them weren't so good, including the time he made her have sex with another man when they were both high and he watched. As the call continues, she begins to lose her patience and grows more anxious about getting back her card.

ALEX: Unspoken but legible on her face is that her sobriety is new, valuable, and precarious. Seeing him, as her words and delivery make clear, would put her new and hard-fought health in danger. But there doesn't seem to be any other options if she is to move forward into rehab.

TED: Again. Back to black. We are left mid-conflict, questions churning in our bellies. Our own experiences, similar to those expressed on the screen, may begin to surface in our minds.

ALEX: Cut to the second scene of this vignette.

TED: The now-familiar furniture has been rearranged yet again, this time to look like a different living room. The camera opens on lines of coke on a table. The actress enters, now out of the shelter and at Spike's apartment. She is wearing a cap and looks cool. He asks her to take a hit of the drugs and she declines: "I told you I ain't get high no more." He responds, "That mean you don't want to have nothing to do with me at all? I sure want to get with you." He is aggravated, jealous, and demanding. He grabs her and begins to kiss her aggressively. She repeatedly asks him to stop. He continues, moans, grabs her

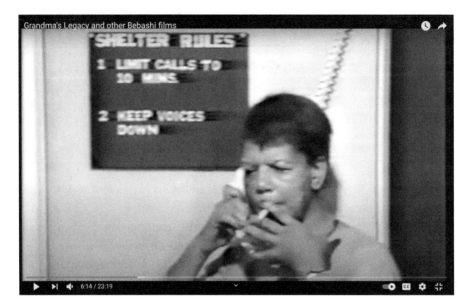

SHELTER RULES
1. LIMIT CALLS TO 10 MINS
2. KEEP VOICES DOWN

6:14 / 23:19

1.3 The second vignette, "Final Decision."

crotch. The camera pulls back to drugs on the table and the scene fades to black, shutting down an unpleasant embrace.

ALEX: Then, within the stillness of the screen, following after the last scene and before any new visuals, from far outside the world of the vignettes something startling, disorienting, and kind of disturbing—in a different register—happens. From inside the blackness of the fade-out you hear the lingering sounds of Spike's arousal: "Ah . . . yeah . . ." The vignette is closing on sounds of his pleasure at her quiet expense. But then, unexpectedly, something else bleeds into and over his moans. We hear the voice of a woman. Firm, brisk, in control: "CUT!"

I love this DIY realness, a new kind of tapey truth. Another assertion of female authority, this time from outside the scene's frame yet inside our screen, seamlessly connects to the previous two stories of Black women also preserved on this video who are attempting to navigate power and authority over their own lives. I choose to read this insertion of a female directorial voice as an intended intrusion that serves as an entree into the third and final scenario, "Grandma's Legacy." But intentional or not, it is an example of the power as well as the messiness of this video, the power of the mess-

24

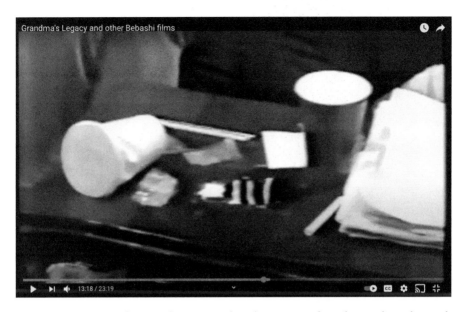

13:18 / 23:19

1.4 The second vignette ends with a pan away from the couple on the couch to a table with drugs. The sound continues to roll.

iness of community-based video: where activism, art, education, and self-representation share one low-budget high-impact frame. And this is much more than enough; it's going to take us pages to unpack!

TED: I didn't notice any outside voice the first time I watched the tape, Alex. But after you pointed it out, I too became intoxicated by that sound. It offered me a new layer through which to experience the video and the women—their authority in places of duress—and also a valuable transition out of the tight hard world depicted over just a few short minutes. It flags that what we are now about to see, the final scene, will be different. And this proves to be the case. We see the same actress from the previous vignette, but she has transformed. It is not clear if she is playing the same character again. Her hair is no longer straight, and it is a different color. Even the quality of the tape suggests that maybe a different camera was used, or that at least there is a new lighting set up.

ALEX: The mood is less brash and more contemplative. The viewer is prompted to think differently about what she sees: perhaps in a less literal fashion. While this vignette is also about illness, risk, and death it is also ex-

25

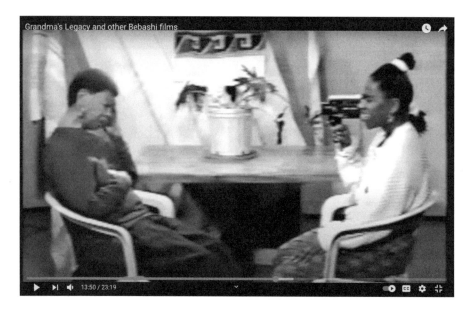

1.5 The final vignette, "Grandma's Legacy," Keisha and Miriam Bennett.

pressly about video, how self-representation and documentation are an integral part of the scene. The establishing shot is of two women; one is holding a video camera. Violent men no longer dominate or even enter the scene. Instead, seated across a table from the actress we recognize from the previous story is another Black actress, much younger. She is holding the video camera. (Was it her voice that said "cut?") We learn her name is Keisha; she is the daughter in this scenario. She delivers the scene's first line: "Hey, this is deep. It's working. Okay, okay, I gotcha now." As she speaks, the point of view switches from the establishing shot of the two women together. The two cameras (hers and the unseen, second one that is taping her filming) are now serving as an intergenerational bridge, much as this video is a bridge between you and me, Ted. We see a blurred close-up on the older woman's face as it comes into focus, as if from the perspective of Keisha's camera: she's attending with a keen tenderness—again, much as we are now—to the stories, words, needs, and problems of this one Black woman in crisis, in Philadelphia, in the late 1980s. The perspective switches once again and we see Keisha as she says: "Come on, Mama. Say something please, we said we'd do this for the kids."

TED: The mother and daughter have come together to shoot a video interview using the daughter's new camera—an expensive but necessary indulgence that we learn through their dialogue cost $900.

ALEX: That was a lot of money for this family and that time! The consumer-grade quasi-professional camcorder that I bought for my own community-based AIDS educational video project, WAVE (the Women's AIDS Video Enterprise, 1990), cost just that, but I bought mine with a $25,000 grant from the New York State Council for the Humanities.

TED: In this case too, a precious video camera will capture this story for posterity. She begins with an introduction: "I am Miriam Bennett and I am thirty-eight years old, although I am sure I don't look it right now." She goes on to explain that she has AIDS and is not sure she will live long enough to meet her grandchild and pass on her legacy in person.

ALEX: The final scenario is her lengthy presentation of her past focusing on AIDS: a complex story dealing with death as well as survival, and the sharing of secrets about brutality against women and girls that underlie her family, sex life, and illness. It uses video, and the doubled act of taping and generation-saving we've already noted, as a catalyst for hard conversations between many groups of people: the mother and daughter in the present of the story; the fictional progeny in the video's future; the actual intended viewers of the educational tape by Bebashi in the 1980s, women from urban Black communities like the one depicted in the scenarios; and now us, a different, perhaps unimagined if maybe also hoped for viewership in the future.

TED: We learn that Ms. Bennett is living with HIV, but had only become aware of her status after she was "hit by a white guy on the road." She hoped to be able to turn the accident into a financial settlement from which she could at last buy a house for her family. But instead of a final legacy of domestic security, she is having to plan for her death.

ALEX: And as if this isn't enough, as this sequence plays out we learn that she contracted HIV from an abusive lover, Bill, who she had caught trying to rape Keisha when she was a little girl. If the previous two vignettes seemed hard, there is even more pain animating this one. It is thick with layers of tragedy and violence, but also hopes for connection.

TED: And with this last scene we find an echo of the first, a mother doing what she can to protect her child. In the first vignette, the mother scoops

27

her child off-screen and attempts to shift the man's mood by using sex. In the second vignette, a viewer may have hoped that after enduring Spike's advances the woman will get her card, and be on her way to further stability. In this final scene, the (grand)mother describes yet more courses of action in relation to domineering men: one of her responses to his violence will prove to be violent itself. When she became aware of Bill he was already on Keisha, and so she needed to spring into action; she knifed him several times to stop him. The police were called. As he was being taken away to jail, she learns from him that he has been sleeping with other women, repeatedly.

ALEX: It is a brutal story to witness in its telling. But this taped witnessing is her second empowering response to abuse. The grandmother delivers her story staccato between sobs. Her last line is a lament, less about dying of AIDS and more about the injustice of having survived so much, including getting hit by a car that she thought would be a ticket out of poverty. Her words:

> Who would have thought that I would be dying of AIDS. Ain't that the shit. I get my ass kicked for six years, barely save my child from a rapist, move out, finally get my life together, and the minute I get a case to haul off, and I be dying.

TED: The scene ends with Ms. Bennett burying her face in her hands and with both women crying as Keisha calls out, "Mama . . . Mama." In my chest I feel heat rise up and my face goes wet and red. While the screen fades to black again, for me, feelings are left very vivid. And on your VHS dub of the vignettes, the sound and the image cut off here together. There is another quick dip to black and a flurry of grey static before the screen goes, at last, to VHS blue. The word "PLAY" appears in the right lower corner. This is a fitting conclusion: an invitation to stop, shake your head, take a deep breath, look around, and begin to make sense of all that was just seen.

28

TRIGGER 1
WHAT WE SEE

1 **VIEW AND DESCRIBE**
We have uploaded the Bebashi video online (https://www.youtube
.com/watch?v=jaxGoZqhYtE). When screened together, the three
vignettes are thirty minutes long. Describe what you see, ideally with
someone else.

2 **READ**
Here are three articles from AIDS Crisis Culture about AIDS activist
video:
- Ray Navarro and Catherine Saalfield. "Not Just Black and White:
  AIDS Media and People of Color." *Independent* (July 1989), 18–23.
- John Greyson. "Strategic Compromises: AIDS and Alternative
  Video Practices." In *Re-imaging America: The Arts of Social Change*,
  edited by Mark O'Brien and Craig Little, 60–74. Philadelphia, PA:
  New Society, 1990.
- Frances Negron-Muntaner. "The Ethics of Community Media:
  A Filmmaker Confronts the Contradictions of Producing Media
  about and for a Community Where She Is Both an Insider and Out-
  sider." *Independent* (May 1991), 20–24.

3 **WATCH**
Here are tapes that were made at around the same time:
- *The Colour of Immunity*. Produced for Toronto Living with AIDS,
  1991. AIDS Activist History. Accessed November 14, 2021. https://
  aidsactivisthistory.ca/2017/11/27/from-the-video-vault-the-colour
  -of-immunity-1991/.
- The videos of Carol Leigh, Scarlot Harlot. Accessed November 14,
  2021. http://scarlotharlot.com.

TRIGGER 2
SEEING TAPE IN TIME

TED: Big breath.

ALEX: The Bebashi tape is messy, intimate, intense, and collaborative, not only in terms of its style but also in that it's about so many things at once: gender, race, money, urban America, sexuality and sex, and also performance and video techniques. Central to our thinking about AIDS history, archives, and the present is holding together many different possible lenses that might be useful to read, encounter, or see any piece of AIDS cultural production. We start with an understanding that our needs and wants of AIDS, and its media, change through time, place, people, and community.

TED: To put the tape in historical context, by the time Bebashi was producing this tape in the late 80s or early 90s, there had already been considerable knowledge-sharing on HIV/AIDS, at least at the community level.

ALEX: For example, activists were not convinced that testing was effective.[1] We believed that testing led to possible state surveillance but no possible treatment, or anything close to a cure.

TED: At this time, a diagnosis was often considered a death sentence, a confirmation that premature death was likely imminent.

ALEX: And then, of course, with hindsight we also know that some people diagnosed with AIDS before 1996 did end up surviving, living past their own presumed time stamp.

TED: "Bonus Life" is what my friend—and activist and artist—Jessica Whitbread calls her life after she turned forty, a year she thought she would never see as a person living with HIV.[2]

ALEX: Yes, many of these long-term survivors are with us, people with HIV in their bodies for decades. These are our friends, our allies, and many of them have needs more closely associated to aging than AIDS. There is an important, building, and diverse body of cultural production about, by, and often also for longtime survivors. Of course, these members of our community are diverse, and their needs are specific: as women, or trans people, or Africans, or gay men.

TED: Increasing diversity within representation has always been a goal within AIDS activism and art. When the Bebashi tape was made, while AIDS was being reported on with some consistency in the mainstream press, the impact of race and gender on HIV was not being carefully explored.

ALEX: So much of the Bebashi work, as well as the AIDS activism I was a part of at the time, was about honoring people in the room: where they come from, how they feel good and known, what pushes their buttons. And the work from there was: How did we get to the screen, how do we get others to join us there, what others, what are the ways to help those viewers to interact with what is there? How can video foster more conversation? This is why I was so moved before the last vignette on the Bebashi tape when we hear an unseen and never-identified woman saying "Cut."

TED: I understand the first part of what you are saying, but I am not sure I understand why video matters so much. Or maybe I should say, what role did video play in this work?

ALEX: Video is a mechanism, a method, a machine, a conduit, a practice, an ethics, a record. In this tape, this becomes most reflexively evident when the tape cuts, as the off-screen voice instructs, to the image of a camera in Keisha's hand (a fictional but seen Black woman director) and then to a conversation between the two characters about the power of tape. This brings to a conclusion the composite tape that holds three honest conversations, two of which are not quite so self-referential. With the off-screen voice, and then with the vignette about videomaking on-screen, the uncredited videomakers reveal many of the machines and processes that were integral parts of their larger project of saving, healing, connecting, and discussing the experiences of low-income urban Black women and women of color at the onset

31

of the onslaught of AIDS within their lives, families, homes, and communities. With technology and within community, the videomakers could express themselves, ask questions, educate, and create systems of support that they need. And even more, these can track forward when we push play again now!

TED: So the video, along with being a process of creation, is also a process of reception. It is a document that invites viewers to meet the women on-screen, while also providing an opportunity to be self-reflexive about themselves as viewers and women as they relate to the stories being told. If I have this right, then I think it is interesting to connect the self-reflexive practices of the Bebashi tape to the Denver Principles, which were written before the tape was made at the beginnings of an organized self-health movement within HIV/AIDS. This is a document that came out of a 1983 meeting of people living with HIV at a Lesbian and Gay health conference—including voices like Michael Callen, Richard Berkowitz, and Bobbi Campbell—in which they pushed back against how they were being represented in mainstream media.

ALEX: We are talking here about the often dehumanizing footage that became and stayed ubiquitous on the nightly news: images of white, usually gay men, wasting away, the hunger of the camera picking up only the violence of their Kaposi sarcoma lesions and sores.

TED: Yes, that footage, and also the language and ideology that went with it. In the Denver Principles the group writes, "We condemn attempts to label us as 'victims,' a term which implies defeat, and we are only occasionally 'patients,' a term which implies passivity, helplessness, and dependence upon the care of others. We are 'People With AIDS.'"[3] In the Principles, you have a group of people living with HIV who assert that they do not want to be known first by an ailment, or a status that their ailment might render onto them: victims, or even patients.

ALEX: So much early AIDS work was about defining representation, asserting the humanity and diversity we all knew and were experiencing within the movement.

TED: And this work, I think, was for and by community.

ALEX: We had an interest in and commitment to each other and ourselves. My first AIDS activist video, *Living with AIDS: Women and AIDS*, made with Jean Carlomusto in 1987 for GMHC's *Living with AIDS* cable television show, was about an almost uncovered topic at that time. I set out to conduct research about women's relationship to the crisis within the lively, enraged, burgeon-

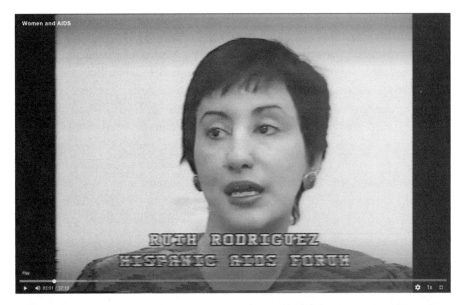

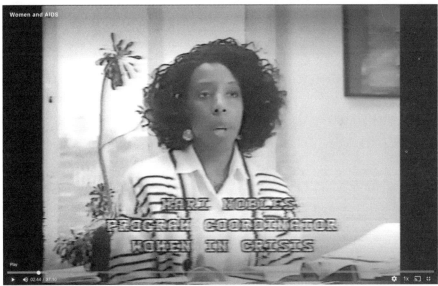

2.1 + 2.2 Screen grabs from *Living with* AIDS: *Women and* AIDS, by Alexandra Juhasz and Jean Carlomusto (1987).

ing AIDS activist and nonprofit scene in New York City. At the time I was not "qualified" in videomaking. I basically lied to Jean about my experience to secure the opportunity. The documentary grew from a shared and developing analysis of newly constituting experts in how to think about women and AIDS. This was being spoken within a real-time cultural, political, and media context and inside a feminist community. Until we did this, women were not understood to really be part of the picture. So maybe I did not know how to make a tape, but we were all learning ways we could analyze, understand, and contribute together. What I did know how to do was reach out, listen, record, and share. And I engaged through a commitment and orientation already developed (if still youthful) from my feminist education in college: to allow women, lesbians, and women of color to be the authorities about our own lives, bodies, and health. Making an intersectional feminist video about AIDS was exactly the right thing to do at the time, in that community, and for me.

TED: Were you worried, though, about your lack of video experience?

ALEX: It didn't dawn on me to *not* make a video about AIDS and women through the lens of intersectional feminism and GMHC'S basic equipment. In this powerful set of approaches and tools, the Bebashi videomakers and many others were fundamentally connected. For me, in New York, there was a community of people around to support this work, speak in the video about this, and eventually view it. Outside of the feminist, lesbian, and BIPOC AIDS activist community which I began circulating in, I was also a member of ACT UP, where video was being actively engaged, and a student at the Whitney Independent Study Program where AIDS activism, analysis, and art was the very air I breathed.[4] *Women and AIDS*, as early as it was, marks and celebrates that there were always worlds of women doing and saying vital things about women and AIDS; that AIDS existed and exists for women; that gender altered and alters the experiences and understandings of AIDS; and that a feminist, anti-racist analysis was best suited to this approach because AIDS has always been disproportionately apportioned to communities of color.

TED: I hear what you are saying about specificity. Who is talking matters, who is behind the camera matters. I get that. Are you also saying that video does something special?

ALEX: Videotape is a conduit for conversation that can lead to transformation. Video lets people do and see and say and share and hear themselves and others in all their beauty and difference. Video helps us to remember who we were as well as giving us things that we need now. We made video at that time because it was our technology during the early days of AIDS Crisis Culture. We can have this conversation now because the Bebeshi video has helped us in a myriad of ways by holding and also triggering memories, histories, processes, analyses, and opportunities for our own transformation.

TED: So something like the Denver Principles is an assertion around how the media and the general public could and ought to engage in the conversation with HIV. And tapes, like the ones made by Bebashi and GMHC, are one animation of the Principles, and their own articulation of related principles of how to view, understand, and see one's self in relation to HIV?

ALEX: Sure. If and when women and people of color were represented as part of the AIDS crisis, they were often blamed for their own infection, or for infecting men. That's why in *Women and AIDS*, we dedicated a good portion of our analysis to distilling the tropes through which women's experience with AIDS were represented, that is when and if women were represented at all: either as "innocent victims," or as vectors. Women who are sex workers have been unfairly blamed, stigmatized, and criminalized as erroneous links to infection. For this reason, starting in AIDS Crisis Culture, connections between prostitute's rights and AIDS activism have been a critical part of AIDS cultural production, informing a feminist analysis of AIDS that centers women's agency, experience, pleasure, and vulnerability. *Women and AIDS* and Carol Leigh's *Safe Sex Slut* (1987; one of many of her AIDS tapes recommended for viewing in the trigger for chapter 1), just like the Bebashi tape, are feminist AIDS work not just because of what they are about (*Women and AIDS* is one of the first videos about this issue), or who we put on-screen (only women are seen as experts in these tapes, and these are predominantly women of color), but also because of the tapes' processes and intentions.

TED: Can we talk about the GMHC audio-visual department in terms of process and intention? That seems like one critical context for understanding AIDS video at this time.

ALEX: Sure. What do you want to know? Jean Carlomusto was hired in 1987 to direct the Audio-Visual Department at the still-fledgling GMHC. After that, Jean collaborated with a generation of makers, committed to cultivating knowledge about the virus by using video. I am proud to say I am part of that community. Many artists and activists collaborated with her including Gregg Bordowitz, who also codirected the unit (and there were many others, like my friends and colleagues Chas Brack, Alisa Lebow, and Juanita

35

Mohammed Szczepanski). They produced the *Living with AIDS* show, which ran on local cable starting around 1987 and continuing until 1996. They also made stand-alone tapes. Many of these are in the Royal S. Marks AIDS Activist Videotape Collection, curated by Jim Hubbard, and archived at the New York Public Library.

TED: I love that an AIDS service organization had a video department headed by someone like Jean, who was cultivating what we could call a feminist, queer, community-based practice of making and distributing AIDS activist video. It helps disrupt this idea of a media desert when it comes to HIV, or an AIDS representational history that is populated only by gay white men.

I also know from Cathy Cohen's work, *The Boundaries of Blackness* (1999),[5] that in the same period that the Bebashi vignettes were being made and disseminated, the mainstream media in the United States was negligent in AIDS coverage. Within that lack, there was a huge disparity in who was covered. In their research, Cohen and her students found that from 1981 to 1993, only 5 percent of the *New York Times* AIDS coverage concerned Black people, and the majority of that was centered around the news that Magic Johnson and Arthur Ashe were living with HIV. They also found that when women were covered in press related to HIV, it was either to position them as victims who were tricked by lying, cheating men, or vectors themselves who people should watch out for, as you have already mentioned.

ALEX: Yes, this research had important effects for activists and scholars. Cohen was just one of that active feminist community of scholars and activists I mentioned above. We were all trying to figure this out together and in real time. Her research helped in so many ways: for instance, how to understand what we needed to do better, what we needed to correct, change, remake. But we already knew what wasn't there; what wasn't seen; who didn't speak in media. That's why camcorders felt so revolutionary at the time. For the first time in history making media began to feel approachable, accessible, affordable, and useful for all those who fell outside the attention of dominant media. Ellen Spiro (like so many others) wrote a manifesto about this: "What to Wear on Your *Video* Activist Outing (Because the Whole World Is Watching)."[6]

TED: It is impressive, and fascinating to realize that at the same time that the *New York Times* was neglecting Black women living with HIV, Black women were leading and founding AIDS responses in their own communities, and making activist videos and other interventions. There was so much work going on, and yet there was no mainstream coverage.

36

ALEX: It's important to remember that even as there was no internet, we always have had an alternative media pressing against these absences and distortions. At this time, Ellen Spiro and others from DIVA TV were partnering with DiAna DiAna and Dr. Bambi Sumpter to make a video, *Diana's Hair Ego* (1991), about the educating and organizing they were doing in Black female communities in South Carolina. There was next to nothing happening there otherwise. So Cohen's research on the lack of reporting on HIV/AIDS and women of color in the *New York Times* is critical. It is one key framework and context for our understanding of the Bebashi tape, particularly as it presses against, or puts into focus, the very activity that was going on in the community as a direct result of and despite invisibility within dominant media. Another instance was at the Brooklyn AIDS Task Force, where I would make the video *We Care* in 1990 within a collective of poor and working-class women of color, and under the supervision of Haitian American AIDS educator Yannick Durrand, who produced videos of her own.

Of course the *New York Times* was negligent, as was ABC, NBC, CBS, and the government. But those dominant media broadcasters are not the only media game in town. For those of us from neglected communities, mainstream media weren't really trusted or accessible sources for information anyway. So building on their scant, bigoted, and judgmental representations so as to diversify knowledge dissemination and better educate communities using their own vernaculars was, in large part, what we were doing with our camcorders. AIDS activist media politics was, to a significant degree, about correcting and augmenting the criminally bad messaging and underreporting of this era.

Critically, our activist efforts were also about moving away from or against an idea of neglect or lack, and instead toward empowerment and creation. We definitely understood—long before Friendster, Myspace, Facebook, Twitter, and TikTok—that we, too, were the media. So even though a place like the *New York Times* may get called "the paper of record," we knew it was important that people understood they had choices when it came to media consumption (and production!) outside of what the government authorized, or what CBS shared. One such tactic, much more common and easy today, was to record and pass on our own knowledge, stories, and experiences. Back in the day that meant making a tape and delivering it into the hands of viewers, programmers, or distributors. Today that means something as quick-to-pull-off as an Instagram story. In either case, the message remains: we were our own (and only) best recorders.

37

TED: I guess it is funny how people can talk about the radicalness of AIDS activism and then still look at a place like the *Times* as a source.

ALEX: But that happens to this day. When scholars or everyday folks talk about AIDS culture it's almost always Hollywood films, or broadcast television, Broadway plays, or marquee art shows. And that's to be understood. Alternative media, radical art, community-based interventions run outside of, in opposition to, and in their own conversations with mainstream practices. This explains how deep we have to look, and with how many interrelated and co-constitutive strategies—high and low, present and invisible, lost and found—to be best prepared to locate our own intersectional, radical, and activist past. This is why we are and need an activist community. We each build one part of the response, and learn from each other as we go. Given that we know that AIDS activism came out of an inadequate response from the government and other dominant institutions, like the media or mainstream culture, then why would those be the only or primary sources we go to for information about the past (or the present for that matter!)? To put "Grandma's Legacy" and the other vignettes in context, we need archival methods as diverse, intersectional, radical, and activist as are our multisited sources.

TED: That makes sense. We can ask ourselves: Will an authoritative voice be the best record of a radical past?

ALEX: Yes indeed, if we are hoping to learn from absences and mistakes and violence.

TED: This impacts how we understand the vignettes in the tape and AIDS media in general. Regardless of whether someone is working on AIDS or not, I think people take media for granted, as if it is one thing: one big thing. Embedded in how we speak about media is this idea that there is mainstream culture and then, over there, somewhere, an alternative culture with nothing in between. Some days I am just happy if people are aware that mainstream culture is not culture in totality. Ha! #amiright

ALEX: Oh Ted, #lowbar. Maybe you need to up your standards. I think if someone is doing work in AIDS cultural production they already understand, as a point of entry, that AIDS will not be the story of the above-the-fold headline, the lead on the nightly news, or the main attraction on the theater marquee. People in specific, local, or political communities understand the ways that mainstream media minimizes, misses, or maligns them and their worlds and issues. So learning from many contemporary and past media scholars, I'd rather situate this and others activist work within a *media ecology*, where individual tapes live within a field of interrelated representation—of different scope, purpose, reach, and orbits—that together define what we know, don't know, and might know.

TED: Oh, I like this idea of a media ecology. It gets us away from monolithic, binary, or dismissive thinking. And it imbues media with a life force of its own, one that reminds us that media is not stationary; it changes over time and within ideas of mainstream, not mainstream, alternative, not alternative, and other designations. There are rich and multiple media contacts, overlays, relationships. I love this notion of us swimming in this infinite body of words, images, sounds, ideas we can call the media ecology.

ALEX: Swimming and producing and consuming and excreting! Media is not stagnant, nor are the people who use and make it. Information—and yes, even life—flows through our fertile and diverse media ecologies.

TED: Right, so to bring it back to AIDS coverage during AIDS Crisis Culture, there was not only the *New York Times*, but also gay newspapers like the *New York Native*, and AIDS-specific alternatives produced in great numbers, like the *Critical Path AIDS Newsletter* or *Diseased Pariah News*.

ALEX: And the hundreds of videotapes about which I wrote my dissertation.[7]

TED: Along with posters, pamphlets, flyers, visual art, performance, support groups, phone trees, activist meetings, and more.

ALEX: A living, vital, self-supporting, if small, messy, underfunded, under-saved, underremembered network that continues to be attended to by a small handful of scholars and activists committed to research about AIDS cultural production. When we explore the AIDS media landscape through the lens of an ecology rather than a monolith or even a binary, we make space for more people to be seen, more work to be acknowledged, and a greater variety of strategies to move past AIDS work carefully forward. And for me, this is personal. We AIDS activist videomakers were all involved in what we understood as alternative media, in its many forms and formats. During this period, trying to make sense of the diverse AIDS cultural production that surrounded him, John Greyson deduced, programmed from, and published a list of many types of tape. It's as useful now as it was then.[8] He didn't call this a "media ecology of AIDS," but he was already flagging how much media there was, how diverse it was, and how interconnected were these many approaches.

But most critically, our place in the ecology was never an alternative to us; it was our world. If anything, the *New York Times* or network TV, with their bad politics and limited, stupid points of view, were the alternative. At the time, Timothy Landers wanted us to be proud of our status as "anti-bodies."[9] For Landers, bodies were "regular" people: straight, white, middle-class, without HIV. Anti-bodies were gay, or Black, or drug users, all us others with AIDS. Bodies are seen all the time; anti-bodies, not so much. Or only in punishing, demeaning ways. We activist mediamakers were (and are) proud to be the anti-bodies, those connected to AIDS and outside of the normalizing forces of mainstream modalities.

TED: How did you register your pride? To each other? To your communities? To the larger public?

ALEX: I'd say it was mostly internal to our small groups of care, activism, and artmaking. Every once and awhile, we'd seek larger audiences. But mostly, those were unavailable. Instead, we were our own best cocreators, community, and audience. We were making friendships and art, flirting, learning, and participating in a vital community, reaching outside comfort zones, and embracing the latest technologies for amazing purposes, all the while sporting our vintage frocks with a head of dark hair, now very gray, as you know. Mine was not that different from the community that formed around the Bebashi tape.

TED: True. As Bebashi's founding executive director, Rashidah Abdul-Khabeer shared with me, when we spoke in July 2020,[10] that the making of the tape was a lot like the third scene in "Grandma's Legacy": Keisha behind the camera, part of the story, but also asking the questions. Bebashi social workers began the process for making their tape with a draft script, but the video was written, taped, and acted by volunteers who were also accessing services at Bebashi.

ALEX: Community-created.

TED: Yes, and as Abdul-Khabeer shared over Zoom, the process they used to make the video was not dissimilar from how they approached other parts of their work at Bebashi:

> Even the Bebashi brochures at the time were done by us. We wrote them and then my sons who were six and eight read them and if they could recite back to me or to our little group what the meaning of those things were then we used them. We consider that functionally

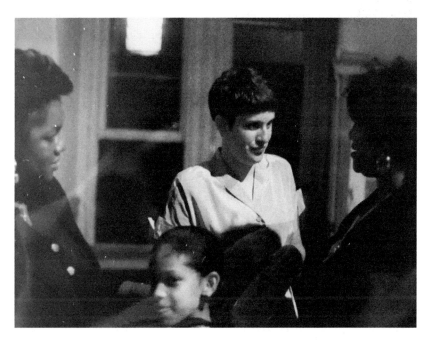

2.3 Downtown Community Television premiere of *We Care* (WAVE, 1990).
From left to right: WAVE collective members Marcia, Alex, and Juanita. Up front,
a young Jazzy, the daughter of Juanita Mohammed Szczepanski.

literate. So if they could understand it then it worked. Those were the
early, nonsophisticated methodologies of really trying to engage the
community in understanding HIV and prevention.

ALEX: That makes sense. As you can see in my photo, when you are working
in community with women, kids are present. They are alive in the room.
They are part of the process. We do our work with and for them.

TED: Bebashi was founded in 1985 by Abdul-Khabeer and Wesley Anderson
when they both worked for the city's Health Department. They were concerned by who was being left behind when it came to AIDS: specifically Black
men, Black people who did drugs, Black women and their children. While the
organization's official title is now Bebashi: Transition to Hope, initially the
name was an acronym: Blacks Educating Blacks about Sexual Health Issues.

ALEX: The tape we are considering is a record of Black women who were not
left behind.

TED: In her work as a nurse for the city, Abdul-Khabeer knew that Black women, marginalized in healthcare settings for their race, as well as their perceived or real relationship to drugs, poverty, and sex work, were being coerced into considering sterilization. They were often made to feel that they had to choose between seeking care for their baby or themselves. That is why from early on Bebashi started to partner with the Family Planning Council to offer wrap-around services for women so they did not have to choose where to get the care they needed. This eventually grew to include five community groups and took on the name Circle of Care.

ALEX: Their feminist intersectional approach is clear in the tape. The context of AIDS in this community was one where female bodies are at risk. It is not until the third vignette, "Grandma's Legacy," that AIDS is even mentioned.

TED: Right! Something I didn't get a chance to talk to Abdul-Khabeer about in our Zoom chat, but comes out loud and clear in Dan Royles's chapter about Bebashi in his book about Black AIDS activism,[11] is that the organization's intersectionality came from the ground up. Staff, volunteers, and people who accessed services were enmeshed in the world of parenting, intergenerational care, sex work, and drug use. Royles points out that this meant that Bebashi staff had "entree into places that other health workers could not."[12] I bring this up because I think it highlights for us, and other viewers of the tape, that for the women we see in the video, HIV was deeply embedded in their lives, and so in hindsight all the vignettes are "about" HIV, not just the last one, which is explicitly so. And of course, that vignette is also about everything that came before and leads to it, including poverty, patriarchal violence, and women's love and need for the men in their lives. Does that make sense? I think about poet and playwright Timothy DuWhite. He speaks about how when it comes to looking for AIDS within Black cultural production, you need to look beyond the surface. AIDS is always there, implicit, and inextricable. I understand him to be saying that this is basically a form of harm reduction. If a viewer needs to see or make connections to HIV/AIDS, they are there for the taking. If someone is not ready, that is okay too.

ALEX: There is a rich, variegated network of trouble through which HIV becomes interwoven into people's lives. AIDS was, from the very start, what people now call a very "intersectional" issue, and as such, impacted communities responded accordingly. There was no other way to approach women.

42

TED: I want to talk about intersectionality as it sits within the media ecology of AIDS. It is important to think about how work was being made in relation to what else was circulating, but some of this AIDS work was not necessarily aware of the other things being made. Does that make sense?

ALEX: Totally. Something worth noting is that the Philly that Bebashi depicts is never seen in the much more viewed AIDS movie, *Philadelphia* (Jonathan Demme, 1993), which would be released only a few years later. I wonder if Demme screened the Bebashi tape as part of his research? *Philadelphia* is a movie about professional people, a white gay man and his Black lawyer, and their experiences of HIV. Where are the Black women living with HIV? The Philadelphians dealing with poverty and HIV? And while I am not interested in disparaging the good work that this and other early narrative films did to put AIDS onto the larger cultural map, if put into contrast with what we are watching closely here, we can see starkly why all the perspectives within an ecology are needed to understand something as complex as AIDS. The narratives, characters, needs, and analyses of AIDS change when viewed through different cultural contexts, new eyes and hands on cameras, and different anticipated audiences. The Bebashi tape would have been circulating slightly later than some of the more well-known early representations: *An Early Frost* (John Erman, 1985) on NBC, *Longtime Companion* (Norman Rene, 1989) in theaters, *The Normal Heart* on Broadway (1985), and Rock Hudson's death dominating headlines. And as someone with familiarity, Ted, what can you tell me that all these better known works have in common?

TED: Nancy Reagan!

ALEX: Ted! Seriously.

TED: Okay. Okay. They are all primarily about white gay men?

ALEX: Yes, exactly. And this is understandable. As with the *New York Times* headline we mentioned, the CDC first recognized HIV in gay men. Yes, the epidemic has devastated many communities, including those of gay men. At the same time, other communities were being devastated and taking action. The work of Black communities impacted by AIDS or women impacted by AIDS was not being seen as widely. Our work had a reduced reach, by definition. And this will to be more seen, better seen, more richly seen inspires more! Alternative media is not simply a correction, it is an addition. That's why thinking through a media ecology is so critical. There is room for expansion, self-representation, correction, all that. Creating alternative media is one way to access a more honest reflection of one's own experience, one that otherwise goes unseen. This has always been a political and artistic project of

43

oppressed people. Let me make it clear: access to making and seeing alternative media has always been the biggest hurdle.

TED: While the formats change, the impulse is fundamental, whether that be slave narratives or dance forms, feminist poetry, or quilts. Art provides a space to have meaningful and specific conversations that name and consider the material and cultural realities of local and political ways of being alive in the world.

ALEX: That impulse is so stunning and live in the three vignettes. This tape visualizes concerns for some Black women living in an urban setting in the later decades of the twentieth century who are figuring out how to care for themselves, their families, and their communities, while also being concerned for their own safety.

TED: Okay, so with that in mind, I want to bring up something that I saw in "Grandma's Legacy." Can you help me to make sense of some lines I thought were confusing—put them into context? The grandmother tells her story for her unborn grandchild but as critically, for the intended audience. As she does so, Ms. Bennett makes an effort to be very clear that she is not gay, has never done drugs other than pot, and has never knowingly slept with a homosexual man. In this way she is refuting all the assumptions at the time around how someone could be living with HIV but also separating herself from these "taboo" behaviors and disreputable people. On first viewing, I have to admit that I was confused that the grandma needed to spell all this out. Distance herself. I am not interested in labeling her approaches as homophobic or anti–drug use. I know that something more interesting or complex could be going on. But I am not sure what! Can putting tapes in context—as we have been doing in this chapter—help me/us understand that part of the tape?

ALEX: But why are you confused? When watching dated tapes, and especially activist video made from within a specific community, we should try to watch with extra tenderness drawn from our best sense of context. So in this case, let's think about what and who the tape was for. We have suggested that the video was made for community-based screenings for Black women, a community that was not being represented by mainstream media in nuanced or even meaningful ways. And anyone who had come in contact with HIV was understood as a pariah, or anti-body, unless you happened to be living within a community of activists.

44

TED: Okay, I am with you . . . and I am remembering that this was also around the time that Cindy Patton formulated her thinking around how contact with HIV makes someone a "queer" subject, regardless of someone's gender or sexuality.[13]

ALEX: So you are disappeared from the media landscape, and you are tackling a taboo subject around which there is a lot of myth, misinformation, and inaccuracies that could prevent people in your community from getting the information and care they need. Meanwhile you are running a program that serves underrepresented populations in a culturally competent way. What are you going to do?

TED: Well, when you put it that way! You will do what Ms. Bennett as a grandma-to-be does: address the misinformation and distance yourself while using the tools at your disposal to help the people who you are about, people who are otherwise going to be ignored by educational campaigns, media, and other institutions.

ALEX: Exactly! While the grandma's denial of homosexuality may come across as insensitive now (or even homophobic then), it was also a way of expanding the conversation, making space for more people—beyond those already assumed to need to know—to talk about AIDS in their own community. Homophobia within the Black community was being addressed by other artists, like filmmaker Marlon Riggs, and Yannick and a team of activist/ artists in their tape *He Left Me His Strength* (Merle Jawitz, Sherry Busbee, Jo-anne Basinger, Sheila Ward, 1989), about Mildred Pearson, who became an activist in Black communities and church, after the death of her son from AIDS, and then, not much later by my ex-partner, filmmaker Cheryl Dunye, and myself, in *The Watermelon Woman* (1996), also a Philly film.

TED: Okay, so while we may live in a media ecology where there is a plethora of media, the mainstream takes up most of the space, and this is to our detriment. There are huge swaths of people that ignore the diversity of the ecology.

ALEX: Maybe not ignore, Ted, but simply don't or can't know, given many constraints on access.

TED: Okay, for reasons that are also part of the larger context, most people focus only on the mainstream, which is often utterly void of an intersectional analysis specific to people from within marginalized communities, let alone simple documentation of the diversity of American experience.

45

ALEX: This isn't because viewers won't. A significant function of dominant media is how easy it is to receive. It takes effort *not* to see it, just as it takes resources to find or make (or save) alternative media.

TED: In the face of all of this, a group of Black women at Bebashi made a tape to address the intersecting social conditions of their day which included but were not limited to HIV/AIDS. And within that work, because of the dominant representations of AIDS being connected to white gay men being spun by the mainstream media and other dominant institutional forces, the women of Bebashi felt it important to push back and name that they were impacted by AIDS in ways that were not experienced by gay men. Their experiences of AIDS looked and felt different.

ALEX: Nor were they white or middle-class.

TED: And so what we are saying is, a study like Cohen's is critical because it helps us to understand what was and what was not happening within the dominant media landscape of the time.

ALEX: And so many other things . . . the *New York Times* need not be the only voice of authority when it comes to understanding the AIDS crisis. As Cohen herself instructs us about her contemporaneous contribution (1999) to this ongoing attempt to understand, so as to better the experiences of African Americans as one community deeply impacted by AIDS:

> Throughout this project I have never intended to condemn the choices or behavior of any particular group of leaders or organizations, but instead to understand why, when faced with a disease that was threatening, significant amounts of African-Americans, traditional black leaders seemed to be doing nothing, or very little. This task led me to investigate fundamental relationships, between power, action, and status *within* African-American communities. To understand the response to AIDS within African-American communities entails the exploration of the intragroup, as well as intergroup, relationships that structure opportunities and information and that correspondingly influence the responses of groups and communities to crisis.[14]

Black women videomakers from Philadelphia are experts and witnesses conversing and educating intergroup. When we witness their thinking today, this is what Cohen understands as intragroup analysis. Following their con-

46

cerns about AIDS in the late 1980s puts all of the cultural production of HIV into a more complete context—in their time, AIDS Crisis Culture, and our own—just as understanding a more complex ecology allows their work to shine.

TRIGGER 2
SEEING TAPE
IN TIME

1 WATCH

Film and video about Philadelphia from the 1990s:
- *AIDS in the Barrio*. Frances Negron-Muntaner, 1990.
- *Philadelphia*. Jonathan Demme, 1993.
- *The Watermelon Woman*. Cheryl Dunye, 1996.

2 READ

Here are four sources about AIDS, women, and Black America from
various Times of AIDS:
- Cathy Cohen. *The Boundaries of Blackness: AIDS and the Breakdown of
  Black Politics*. Chicago: University of Chicago Press, 1999.
- Michelle Tracy Berger. *Workable Sisterhood: The Political Journey
  of Stigmatized Women*. Princeton, NJ: Princeton University Press,
  2004.
- Linda Villarosa. "America's Hidden HIV Epidemic." *New York Times*,
  June 6, 2017. https://www.nytimes.com/2017/06/06/magazine
  /americas-hidden-hiv-epidemic.html.
- Celeste Watkins-Hayes. *Remaking a Life: How Women Living with HIV/
  AIDS Confront Inequality*. Oakland: University of California Press,
  2019.

TRIGGER 3
BEING
TRIGGERED
TOGETHER

TED: In spite of our research and interviews, the most detailed observations we have found about the Bebashi tapes actually came from the short paragraph you wrote about the tape twenty-five or more years ago in *AIDS TV*, which I read in preparation for this conversation.

ALEX: I didn't read the paragraph again—although I easily could have—for reasons that themselves are definitive of our larger concerns about the burdens of and responsibilities for knowing and passing on AIDS information, particularly by way of cross-generational sharing (which is also a subject of "Grandma's Legacy").

I really do wonder, Ted, must I return to my past every time it is evoked by you or others? People today are interested in looking at a history that I lived, wrote about, and have also discussed over decades. I wonder, what are the costs to me or you if the things that my peers and I have already recorded are then revisited? (This is the subject of Part Two, "Silence.") What are the costs, instead, if these objects or processes go lost? If no one cares? If people care but misconstrue, or bring the words and judgments of today on to works from before that can't quite hold such critiques or needs or terms? Why and also how do we carefully and caringly make, save, share, and revisit?

TED: These are all live questions for us, in our relationship to each other, history, and the Bebashi tape. We are trying to think about and also model ways to do this sensitively; take the time to bring forward, with dignity, a work that might otherwise be lost. In the process, we do not deny the role of the viewer—us—and how we are changed by the tape or the process. We allow our different, even contradictory relations to the past to be part of what we can use to understand the tape, particularly in that there is so little available about it other than what we are making here!

ALEX: This is key. Can we hold this or any similar object, one that is precious to us, with care? Can we hold ourselves, as viewers, and then our anticipated readers to the same standards of engagement? This is a dynamic project where writers, readers, and viewers have to understand ourselves in relationship to each other and objects in a variety of media and Times. This, we suggest and hope to show, maybe counterintuitively brings forward our own humanity, as well as that of the people who made and were represented so long ago. This is how any one tape can function as a transitional object that gives us permission to express ourselves as we relate to the work, and to each other, from across time and in this time.

TED: We save and explore a networked past of self, others, and objects, while creating new objects (like a book) for a future cycle of archiving and retrieval. We hope to do this humanely, transparently, and with humility and appreciation.

ALEX: And since I am trying to treat myself with the same care that I would give any tape, or you, I am not making myself go back to read a paragraph I wrote when I was twenty-five, mostly because that feels painful for any number of reasons. First, I can't remember most of it, even though I wrote it. But worse, it feels lost or nearly lost. Like no one, even you, has really read it. And that becomes meta really fast, because then one must ask, what is the use of *this* writing, or any writing? Will anyone read this or anything with the care we hope for as writers who have worked so hard? Will it be remembered and useful twenty-five years from now? Or is our work only or mostly for its doing, for its time? Then, there's the self-critical part: maybe it is not remembered because it wasn't good enough.

But even so, this is not to say that I don't want to engage, or consider, or be in conversation. All this pain is worth the possibilities that new encounters might render. After all, after we watched the DVD of the Bebashi tape, I *did* look for the VHS tape. And I successfully located it in a box on a shelf in a holding room in the library at Brooklyn College, where I had donated it, and many like it, to be saved as part of another related research project: VHS Archives.[1]

TED: I get it, and I am grateful to you as a person with a history and a contemporary practice of curiosity and knowledge production.

ALEX: I don't need you to be grateful, Ted. That is not what I am asking for. And if I am honest, what I am saying is a bit overwhelming for me, but also I think at the heart of what we are doing here.

TED: What do you need?

ALEX: I need you to understand that this is not only about me. You also have a past and present. What do you need?

TED: I guess, like you, I need different things. Right now, the most pressing is that I need to understand how best for us to work together to serve the object we are talking about. We have watched the tape, put it in some context, and now we are bringing our own experiences into our reading. So I guess I need to know that we have a process in place that allows us to remember that time is not a line. When we feel confronted, or out of sorts, or hysterical, the conversation and our process can hold us, and the object.

ALEX: Thanks. So let me try again. Not only did I live and work through these times, I had ideas, I wrote them down, and then they were published. And I did this work within a community of other smart and creative people, and we were learning from each other. We figured a lot out, and things were better in our time because of it. I feel good about that. But then, fast-forward a few decades later. Here I am, still a teacher, a writer, and an activist, and I'm still working on AIDS and related cultural and political issues. Now I am frequently in spaces where I see people trying to figure out for themselves, for the first time, things that we knew and said decades earlier.

People are doing their AIDS work now by building on our work, redoing that work, and sometimes with no knowledge of our work. And that is fine, human, a bit confusing, and also a little unsettling.

TED: Right, and maybe there are ways that we are redoing or even overdoing people's work that has already been done. I get that. But let me catch up a bit. I think what you are saying is that part of being in a movement for a long time is having to witness the shifts in understanding and the changing production of culture that then facilitates changes in knowledge—

51

ALEX: Yes, and related practices and experiences in the world! Things change when empowered groups of people (even those on the margins, even small groups of people) make and circulate work with new ideas and demands built from inventive and productive processes.

TED: And for you, there is a sense of unsuredness about how to deal with being that witness, especially while engaged in conversation with someone like me who you consider a peer, but also someone who has different and less experience than you.

ALEX: Yes, but also, I'm both a witness and an actor at the same time. That's disconcerting. These are different and sometimes competing roles. And it's not that you have less experience than me. Just less time on the earth and in our movement. You're a forty-year-old man. You have reams of experience. I started working on AIDS when I was twenty-three!

TED: I also started this work when I was in my early twenties, but in a different mode and time.

ALEX: Earlier, I was vulnerable with you about what this process brings up for me. That is part of the process we are learning and extending from the tape. Now, I'm trying again to give you an opportunity to be humane and careful with me, with this process, with the tape. Take the time to share how you feel, or name what you need in this process.

TED: I guess I need time and space to figure out my feelings about our process. To be fair, you have had more time, and maybe even a broader range of experiences in being in this AIDS world, in having texts published, in changing your mind, in forgetting, and being asked to remember. I really get that you are suffering having a book forgotten, but this is my first time writing a book. This is all new to me. So it seems critical to note that while we enter this process with a shared object, the Bebashi tape, and shared questions about AIDS, and a shared set of processes we are developing together to engage—

ALEX: We have different relations to authority and voice and books . . .

TED: . . . We should stay mindful about the ways that my past, your past, and our shared present collide or diverge.

ALEX: As well as our needs. You are no more a naive baby than I am a relic, even if I must be an "elder." We are still doing our work in the present, but I just happen to also have adult knowledge (albeit young adult) of a period of great value to our work, as well.

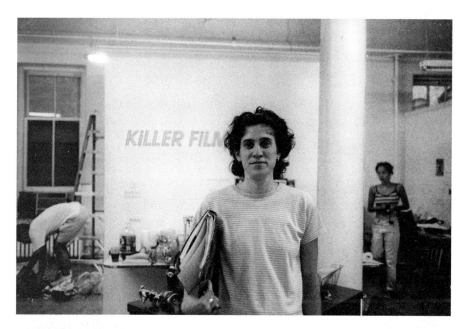

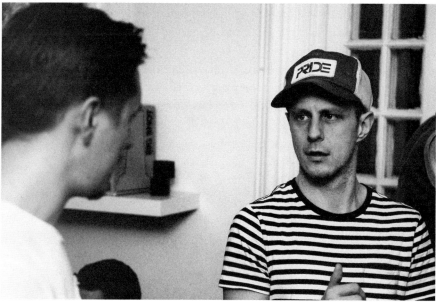

3.1 + 3.2 Alex and Ted, doing their work in New York City in their early thirties. Different decades but similar shirts. Credit: Photographer unknown, and Unusually Fine.

TED: Okay, sometimes we do have to repeat ourselves, even if the echo is two decades coming, or much closer at hand, like the previous chapter . . . This work is hard, and in our interactions we aren't always clear or fully heard on the first pass.

ALEX: And the conversation changes us and what we know. And it's happened over time, and actually not linearly, even if it is presented as such here.

TED: So we can also attest that you finding the VHS dub was helpful. In light of the absence of any title cards on the tape itself, it is actually from your handwriting on the box label that we learned that the scene that makes up the middle vignette is called "Final Decision," and the last one is fittingly called "Grandma's Legacy."

ALEX: This tape was among hundreds that I collected and watched in the late 1980s as part of my doctoral research on AIDS activist video. I was in my late twenties and living in New York. These research materials came to me in a variety of ways: through friends and colleagues who were also AIDS video activists; by reading through mimeographed lists of AIDS video collections built and maintained by nonprofits and public health organizations around the United States for their clients who needed information and insight; from gay and lesbian film festivals where some of this work was screened; and even from the art world where there was a keen interest in activist AIDS arts in certain quarters. My files for my doctoral research are filled with many photocopied lists of video holdings that catalogue collections of AIDS videotapes that were being produced and shared all over the world. Now such lists are online and easier to get to. But the care and time that is registered in the handmade lists is something that goes lost in digital settings.

There were so many of us writing, thinking about, showing, or making AIDS video at this time, inside and outside of academia, as well as in art worlds, nonprofits, health organizations, activist communities, and elsewhere. This large multifaceted movement was the subject of my dissertation, which went on to be my first book, *AIDS TV*. Fast-forward a bit and I got a job and left New York. Like so many who lived, I moved on and became pretty quiet about AIDS. Even so, I lugged these VHS tapes and many more with me when I moved to Los Angeles in 1995 to teach in Claremont, California. Then I brought them back across the country when I moved back to New York City in the summer of 2016 for my new job at CUNY.

TED: Which is when I first had a chance to watch the tape with you, in your then only recently unpacked living room.

ALEX: This was the beginning of our face-to-face working conversations. We had worked together before, but always using phones or computers, and much more as AIDS activist colleagues then as the friends we would become. Now that I was in Brooklyn, and we had become inadvertent neighbors, we began to meet regularly in the domestic space of my home, and this usually included bagels, gossip, and important catch-ups on the sprawling AIDS activist cultural landscape we are both navigating (and cocreating with others) in New York. We were—and are—part of a growing conversation. Today, we still take walks together in our neighborhood and we have traveled together on six or more retreats to write this book!

The possibility for friendship, analysis, and attending together to earlier art and people was first really cemented when I brought out a pile of DVD transfers to share with you. And I have to say what was so cool about this is that it was so similar to my experiences during AIDS Crisis Culture when I was doing AIDS work with friends in our domestic spaces. You and I met on the internet, and wrote our first conversations online and on the phone. The internet has a way of creating conditions for working, but this is usually done alone, in our separate spaces. Somehow, with luck and life changes, our processes—which were growing out of our shared attention to the past—had also pushed us to engage together in the world, using but also without the digital.

TED: It's fun and empowering to work on things that matter to you with trusted conversation partners. But Alex, that also happens online all the time. Because of the internet there can be other kinds of collective experiences of living with illness. Activists who can't leave their apartment, let alone their beds, can coordinate and participate in actions. In Jennifer Brea's 2017 documentary *Unrest*, we see people living with myalgic encephalomyelitis (ME, often referred to as chronic fatigue syndrome [CFS] or ME/CFS) all across the United States using Skype to organize national protests. Some of them are able to attend the protest in the flesh, and others participate from their beds. In fact, Brea herself does many of the interviews for the film from her bedroom.

Community around illness is formed. I also want to mention here the Canaries, a group of women and femmes living with chronic illness who support each other through an online forum and at times shared art practices, like their 2016 residence in New York's Recess space.[2]

ALEX: For sure, the internet—and how it holds and shares video, photography, text, and other media—has expanded and altered our possibilities for

55

the production, sharing, and consumption of both new and old AIDS media, new and legacy AIDS communities, and new formats for memorialization of those lost to AIDS as well as other illnesses and viruses.

TED: Right. And you've experienced and worked within both video and digital technologies across several decades. Your perspective on this is really valuable. But I also know that you often have reservations about how and when to be the person with a past in our conversations. So I often feel a sense of uncertainty about when it is useful for me to question, inquire, or push back on lessons from the past offered by people who lived it. Which is not to say that I am treating you or anyone with kid gloves or choosing deferment over engagement. Rather, there are times when someone will say something that is true to them about a time gone by and will also attempt to apply this knowledge to the present. Then I have to calculate when it is useful for me to talk about the present, or instead, when it is okay for someone to learn something more slowly, over time, and maybe not from me. For example, in this case, while there is truth and power in what you said about what can and can't happen when we are online, at the same time I don't want people reading this book to think that we don't know that there are legions of communities who have a collective understanding of HIV or illness today because of the internet and the ways it allows people to connect and engage.

ALEX: Indeed, as someone whose ongoing work is about striving for queer feminist internet culture, I think about and attend to the movements of activist and once only IRL communities into online spaces. My most significant concern about the changing norms of activist interactions is about how and if they afford for our being together in physical space (and/or shared time), and from that building something new or more.

TED: Right. I think that meaningful and political interactions can happen IRL and digitally.

ALEX: And it can—and must—happen across time. As much as I have a multifaceted relationship to how I want our work from the past to be understood and considered in the present, I don't want the politics and influences of the past to get lost or be conflated with those of today, or to be understood as more (or less) valid. Of course this can happen online or off. And sure, in some ways that's a burden, and a heavy lesson: what you made before is made for its time, to be mostly forgotten, and only maybe to be refound or redone (again). But that is also at the heart of our theory and practice of using conversation as an archival and activist method to learn from the ongoing and

56

past cultural production of AIDS. Capturing, storing, and saving are never enough. It is the connecting, sharing, and changing of objects that matters (to people).

TED: When I teach about AIDS, be it in a university class or a workshop setting, I like to begin with the question "How do we know what we know?" about HIV. This helps to name our lens or bias, and to announce our ignorance as well as our expertise. It is also a good way to think about cultural production: What informed this video or that essay? Where is it coming from? What informed it and also me? And then, What do I or we bring to it? So I appreciate all the various burdens and experiences and ignorances we bring to this conversation, and I actually need to hear them said to really see many of them, for myself as well as for you. And I hope that as we raise both questions and strong ideas for each other about our different pasts and shared present, we do so for the reader as well. I am excited by the ways we are trying to expand this format to engage with our readers in challenging that.

TRIGGER 3
BEING
TRIGGERED
TOGETHER

1 **EXPLORE**

What are careful ways to engage in conversation about our personal AIDS histories? What do you need? What do others need?

2 **WATCH**

Three videos made for Day without Art, "Alternate Endings Radical Beginnings," in which artists and activists engage with their own AIDS objects from the past. Videos can be found at https://visualaids .org/projects/alternate-endings-radical-beginnings.
- Thomas Allen Harris. *About Face: The Evolution of a Black Producer* (2017).
- Cheryl Dunye and Ellen Spiro. *DiAna's Hair Ego REMIX* (2017).
- Kia LaBeija. *Goodnight, Kia* (2017).

3 **READ**

Four books by activists and artists who engage with their own AIDS objects from the past:
- Gregg Bordowitz. *General Idea: Imagevirus*. London: Afterall, 2010.
- Anne-Christine d'Adesky. *The Pox Lover: An Activist's Decade in New York and Paris*. Madison: University of Wisconsin Press, 2017.
- Lyle Ashton Harris. *Today I Shall Judge Nothing That Occurs: Selections from the Ektachrome Archive*. New York: Aperture, 2017.
- Eric Rhein, *Lifelines*. Lexington, KY: Institute 193, 2020.

TRIGGER 4
BEING
TRIGGERED
IN TIMES

ALEX: I hate to break it to you, Ted, after all that great work that we did, but the way that you and I tended to the tape in chapter 1—paying close attention to the actors, camera angles, set, and lighting—was not necessarily the way it was primarily or initially intended to be seen or used. It was not made as an aesthetic or art object, even as it has a very powerful look and feel.

TED: How was it supposed to be watched in its time?

ALEX: It is from a now lost subgenre—the trigger tape—made to be used in educational settings and in therapeutic contexts with trained facilitators. At the time, we thought a lot about the best ways to use video for education and community-based activism. Ray Navarro and Catherine Saalfield's [Gund] writing and activism about this was very impactful. In their work for Media Network in the early 1990s, they created templates for community-based screenings of carefully chosen tapes, which they then shared with other activists and educators in the publication "Seeing through AIDS."[1] We were all thinking about using tapes as a critical part of our AIDS activism. Another example is Catherine Saalfield's [Gund] helpful videography for my book, *AIDS TV*, where she reiterates their theory of "media use." For the book, I commissioned a videography from her that would do more than create a list of tapes. She writes about how each of the tapes she presents on this list can be used, and by whom.[2] Talk about the hard work and multiple registers of loving activism! Her videography, like so many linked interventions, details the care of our community for the objects we had made only quite recently with care. Our videos were made to *trigger* conversation, a word that is still in use. But in a different way.

TED: It is funny to think about how a word that now has become associated—for better or worse—with warning viewers about content, allowing them to decide if they want to opt out of conversation or even looking, was once an invitation for initiating hard-to-have discussions.

ALEX: Silencing was never our thing. We'll spend Part Two, "Silence," trying to make sense of how it did and did not work for us, and how it stays with us. But to begin simply here. Silence equals death, remember?

TED: I. I remember. But trigger warnings are not silencing, are they? Aren't they about providing choice and respecting that trauma is real, something we could argue is as paramount to AIDS activism as "silence = death"?

ALEX: Yes. And because we are respecting current parlance and norms we provided a trigger warning to this trigger tape when we first asked our readers to watch it, in the trigger for chapter I. This is because the three vignettes sit entirely within sites of trauma. In its time, however, a favored way to respond to trauma was to open into it within a supportive environment. To name and see it, together. Today, viewers or users ask for new viewing and healing practices connected to making more overt the potential harms associated with witnessing and visibility in media now that everything is so easy to see, share, and experience, and is usually received in isolation and without context.

TED: Ironically, for a class I taught on AIDS, history, and memorialization, I decided to show "Grandma's Legacy," that is to say just the final vignette, and I failed to include a trigger warning.

ALEX: Ted! How can you be lecturing me about trigger warnings here, and then in your own work with college students you tell me you don't even (remember to) use them!

TED: Wait. It is worse. I normally *do* use trigger warnings, or as I have come to say: content announcements. But for reasons to do with timing and the material I wanted to get through that week, I showed the video in the last twenty minutes in class.

60 ALEX: Wait, so they did not even have time to process the content in class with you before moving on with their day? That is crazy. And wrong! You know better . . . these vignettes are *tough*.

TED: Exactly. And this was the problem.

ALEX: I am sorry, Ted. I can relate. Sometimes we get so excited to share the things we love, and hope that our students or colleagues or friends will love too, that we lose sight of our larger commitments. And yes, sometimes we are just too busy or rushed to be as careful as we know how.

TED: After the tape was over and people were shuffling out of class, one of them slowed down and suggested that I might want to check in on some students before the next class. This was a very kind thing to do, and it echoed with the pit forming in my stomach as I watched "Grandma's Legacy" with an uninitiated audience. While I am still not desensitized to the brutality expressed in the work, it was upon seeing it in the classroom with the students that I realized I had made a mistake.

ALEX: So what did you do?

TED: Within ten minutes, I emailed the class apologizing for not giving them space to process the work. Then, I invited them to contact me to discuss further. One student took me up on the offer. They had found the work so upsetting that they were distracted in their next class that day, which I understood. We met, I apologized in person, we named what could have been done better by me, and then talked about the tape and other related issues. Then, for the next class, I started by naming what had happened, and opened things up for conversation. That was that.

ALEX: Not to get too self-serving here, but talking about talking and not talking is often the best way to trigger a conversation.

It seems like the order of things, as it relates to trigger, has changed. It used to be a function that came after a difficult utterance or image, and now it comes before. Without picking a side in the culture war around triggers, it is instructive for us, given our attempts to engage with objects with respect to their Times, as well as our own, that in the previous incarnation of the word, trigger was paired with conversation. Today it serves as a warning to protect interaction. In both senses—whether you do so at the beginning or end of a conversation—it is a useful method for conversing about how damage sits and moves by way of things made by people before us. Trigger centers care and interaction and exchange.

TED: Yes, but of course, what so often goes unnamed in these trigger conversations is that the word itself is so intense; it can connect to bullets, guns, premature death, police violence, domestic assault, white supremacy, and so much more. Even before we talk about trigger tapes or trigger warnings, the word itself is powerful and imbued with meaning, and sorrow. So as this conversation on the shifting meaning of trigger attempts to be caring and careful, I think we would be wise to be and stay humble, knowing that no amount of theory or explanation or rationale will counter the brutality of the word's connection to life and death.

ALEX: Thanks for adding that here, Ted. The term "trigger tape" is a good example of what happens when we try to dislodge a word from one association while keeping all its associations live. Trigger is also a mechanism, a release of stored energy that upon release has impact. In the case of a gun, trigger is violent, death-dealing, and maim-inducing. When it comes to tape, at least as I and we have experienced it, trigger is about releasing the power of human experience to inspire sharing and connection. In this iteration of the word, trigger is about possibility.

TED: Every generation grapples with their trauma and this can be enabled and helped, but also at times fueled or frustrated by language and technological advances: for instance, today we ask what to do when more information becomes unfettered, or less censored, or more available. I wonder if the influx of possibility is what creates new cultural calls for equilibrium. Keeping one notion of trigger as a mechanism in mind, maybe trigger warnings are as much about the real and often brutal content that now so easily floats past our fields of vision as they are about creating some sort of dam on that content, a warning sound before impact.

ALEX: Unlike the internet culture and media space of today—a world of representational abundance in need of boundaries—the world we were hoping to make or at least see newly in the earlier years of AIDS Crisis Culture, where our medium was VHS video, was organized by an almost complete and just-breaking silence (the First Silence): all those who couldn't or wouldn't speak, who spoke but were barely seen, like the Black female characters we meet in the tape for whom testifying in real life rather than on tape as actors would have been difficult and would have meant certain danger if they pulled it off.

Each one of the testimonies in the tape was meant to be witnessed and also processed as a stand-alone story, and in a context different from, and well outside of, the dangerous homes being depicted. You should "do it on tape," as the Grandma says to her granddaughter at the beginning of section three of the video, precisely because you weren't ready to do it at home. A place that was and is often unsafe for many of us—due to violence, drugs,

62

patriarchal control, and structural racism. A productive screening of the tape attempts to create a different context within which a more considered response to these dangers can take place, not possible during a real crisis. Imagine each scene being played, one at a time, and then stopped at the fade to black. It was not to be watched as we did—as one steady unroll, as if it is one tape rather than three. And the viewing would be in a church basement, community hall, or doctor's office waiting room for a small handful of people, probably women, whose lives may have been quite similar to those depicted on the screen. The end of each scenario is left *un*played because the intention is for the audience, as a community, to help each other play out the characters', and really their own, next steps. In this way, trigger warnings now, and trigger tapes then, are both about attempting to shepherd responses, through invitation or warning, as needed.

At a screening of a trigger tape, after each vignette a facilitator should start a conversation about what has just been seen. The emphasis should be on inviting connections between the scenes and people's lives, feelings, and past experiences. The tapes were made to move audiences into collective understandings about the struggles and realities of their own lives: for example, what is at risk for them personally, in their own homes, when and if they decide to negotiate safer sex with a male lover, partner, or husband.

TED: Right, hence the tape's focus on story, and the lack of information about who made the tape. They knew they made the tape for themselves and other women they knew.

ALEX: When you are your own audience, and the focus is on process, no credits are needed.

TED: I want to say two things about this. First, in Dan Royles book *To Make the Wounded Whole: The African American Struggle about HIV/AIDS* he interviews Bebashi staffer Curtis Wadlington about a trip he took for the organization to Cameroon in which the communities were putting on plays about AIDS for each other. Upon seeing that play he realized that culture was the right place to work with any group made marginal.[3] After reading Royles, I thought about how this trigger tape is as intimate as a play being performed in front of you. Second, I wanted to say that in my chat with Abdul-Khabeer she basically said what you just shared about the lack of need for credits. She explained that the tape "was really designed to talk to the women . . . to help them examine issues of impact, self-empowerment. They were just scripted scenarios so that they could learn to explore and have discussions about it, talk about things so that they can literally visualize it, the things that were happening around them."

ALEX: That is an important reminder. The tape was not really or at least at first made for us, nor for the people that will see the vignettes now that we've put them online.

TED: In sharing the tape, made by and for Black women in Philadelphia during AIDS Crisis Culture, we are inviting alternative viewership and engagement for different but related goals.

ALEX: Which is at the heart of community-based video process. You make something, and you put it out into the world, and it meets audiences and situations you try your best to anticipate and even care for (if that is your media ethic). If those audiences change, rethinking goals is part of the process.

TED: So what is our duty then, upon encounter?

ALEX: Engagement on our terms. Understanding how our needs are aligned, and disparate, from AIDS communities different from our own.

TED: Can a tape like this work outside the space, place, time, and community from whence it came?

ALEX: Want to find out? Are you game to respond to one of the triggers? Play it out?

TED: Out of respect for the trigger process?

ALEX: Yes, but also for the women who made it, and their goals for the tape: to inspire reflection and conversation. As a cis white HIV-negative gay man who has watched the tape, who has been discussing and teaching it, the least you can do is be part of the cycle of vulnerability and sharing.

TED: Will you join in?

ALEX: Of course. As a mostly but not at all times white, upper-middle-class heterosexual woman, one could argue the tape was not made with me in mind either. But I will suggest that our willingness to both identify with and differentiate ourselves from these characters, their time, and their troubles is one example of the conversational processes we are attempting to practice and share. And the trigger helps us in ways different from and similar to what might be expected from how it would have worked with its initial target audience and in its original Time of AIDS.

64

TED: Okay. I am game.

ALEX: Good. Here we go. Episode One ends with the woman in a sexual embrace with her abusive husband having gotten her daughter safely out of the room. We agree that she uses the sexual act primarily as a way to mollify her enraged partner and defuse the danger to herself and her child. First off, and I know this is hard: Have you ever done this? In my sexual history, thank god I've never had a physically abusive male lover who I've had to pacify with sex, but I have had a verbally abusive partner, and I've definitely offered sex to de-escalate. In my sexual and domestic life, I think this sometimes worked well. Sex can change the feelings; remind you both about and bring love back into the equation. Of course, it can also come with resentment, which can and usually does play out later, sometimes as more violence. Would you have diffused this situation with sex?

TED: I will answer, and I am happy to answer. But then I will also double back a bit and name for readers why I think we are doing this exercise.

ALEX: This feels like a stalling attempt, but okay.

TED: So, to the question if I have ever used sex to mollify an abusive lover: yes and no. I have done it to make an unsavory ex go away, and I did sexual things I did not want to do with a man I met online because going through with it was easier—and I will say less dangerous for my personal safety—than not. But I have never been in a relationship with someone who was threatening or violent—emotionally, physically, or sexually.

   Now, for why we are doing this. We are following the lead of the material— that is to say the tape—while also doing what was asked of people who watched the tape in its time. And this is a version of what we are asking our readers to consider doing at the end of each chapter—

ALEX: Which is . . .

TED: Which is to be vulnerable, open, thoughtful, and communicative in a shared environment about tapes, and some of what tapes might trigger.

ALEX: Fear. Love. Questions. Knowledge.

TED: Nostalgia. Grief. Interaction.

ALEX: Okay, so back at it. Given our shared interests, and those of Bebashi, it seems important to talk about whether I would have used a condom in this situation, or whether we think the cis woman in the vignette asked her lover

65

to use one, or should have. My guess is that she did not, and if I was her, I would not, and if I was me, I would not. And this is really hard to talk about (which is why there is a trigger here!). Most straight cis men (and cis women) I know think that HIV is not an issue of relevance; denial, I know. Over the course of my life, I have heard countless men (cis, straight, and queer) complain that condoms affect their performance and pleasure. And while I will only nod to this here, there is a parallel set of concerns within queer couples where a dominant partner can make negotiating around sexual health feel dangerous, as this might be linked to fear or possible abuse. In a common heterosexual dynamic, the man would be dictating the terms of the encounter. In my sexual history I have "negotiated safer sex," but this usually happens well before sex, or to be honest, after a few sexual encounters when the original crazed desire to copulate has evaporated and the chilling truth of danger begins to percolate more noticeably on the surface of interactions. Again, given that I have behaved so "badly," and I have always been super self-chastising about this, particularly because I've been an AIDS activist since I was twenty-three, how would I expect any woman to "do better," given the specter of violence in the room?

TED: There are 100+ things to say here, but I will keep the spirit of the exercise in mind and just say a few: I feel that no one should ever feel judged for using or not using a condom. I feel that so many forces are galvanized to make us feel shame that imposing shame on oneself is not helpful. And yet I also know that people can feel how they want to feel about things they have done in their lives and don't need my permission or anyone else's to feel shame, joy, glee, fear, or whatever.

ALEX: Are you avoiding the condom question?

TED: Me? No! What I just said is part of my answer! Ha. What I can also tell you is, I used condoms when I was young, and that was a period during which the space that the condom put between me and partners was welcome. I was working through a lot of internalized homophobic thoughts about anal sex. Condoms were the equivalent of the holy ghost at high school dances for me. Then, as I got older and worked through my homophobia, I started to realize I don't like using condoms, and me and my partners did not feel it was needed. So I basically stopped using them. All of which is to say, with our example in mind, I am not sure condom use is the thing I would be thinking about. And I say that fully aware that I am a gay cis white man who cannot get pregnant, and for whom receiving an HIV diagnosis would have big impacts, for sure, but would be less of a burden than it would be for so many other people. When it comes to sex, I am almost always more impacted by the risk of emotions.

ALEX: Remember when I called you with an HIV scare when I was still living in California? I had had sex one time with a man I met on the internet. We both moved on. About exactly six months later he called and said he had received an HIV+ test result. We hadn't had safe sex although we had discussed our sense of known risks beforehand. I was frantic. I knew that HIV could be controlled with medication, but I didn't want a diagnosis of a manageable but serious health condition, like diabetes or high blood pressure, because of HIV's stigma, because it meant that the rest of my life would be medicalized, and I thought it would seriously impact, for the negative, my sex life as a single queer woman hoping for connection, sex, intimacy, and honesty with others.

TED: I remember. We spoke on the phone. It was dark out and I was walking in Soho to catch a subway on Canal Street. I stopped to listen under some construction scaffolding. We talked out the very thing you are bringing up right now, the desire to not compound the stigma of HIV through "being dramatic," and the very reasonable desire to not have more complications in your life. It is a hard balance. As someone who has worked to not be afraid of HIV, I am often confronted and confused—be it through my friends' lives or my own—about how to honor the power of HIV with many people's preference to live without it, including those who have it.

ALEX: For many of our friends and colleagues living with HIV, their diagnosis propelled them into community, activism, health, anger, and power. My experiences in conversation with HIV+ friends have been transformative in that I have had to reckon with a complex reckoning with our unique and shared power and vulnerability, difference, distance, and proximity as humans in a world with HIV. As always, for me, when I can be open about my position and can engage in conversation with others who are also trying for openness, I am also most open to being changed.

TED: The tape tries to create a structure like that, Alex. Would it be too obvious to say that rooms of women watching trigger tapes together are analogous to consciousness-raising groups? Both are ritualized spaces in which women and people whose voices are often left unheard come together to share information and build power through exposure, self-empowerment, trust-building, and resource-sharing.

67

ALEX: I don't think it is the same. Consciousness-raising is a specific set of methods and directives refined by the women's movement during second-wave feminism. A group would meet many times over months or even years and the end goal would include direct action or social change projects responsive to a new and shared understanding of one's individual experience, connecting to those that were similar in the group, only then to be understood as a symptom and product of larger structural forces. A trigger tape shown to an audience is by definition a one-off, and the insights and changes anticipated would be primarily in the realm of personal or domestic behavior. That is to say, AIDS educational trigger tapes were less about movement-building and more about personal empowerment and communal recognition.

TED: Okay. That makes sense. When asking the question, I had not considered the durational aspect of a consciousness-raising group. I think now of the Silence = Death collective, which started as a consciousness-raising group for men dealing with HIV in the pre–ACT UP era. They met over months at each other's houses for meals and conversation, and over time they made the choice to make something together, and then share it with the world. For me, the story behind Silence = Death brings even deeper meaning to the iconic image. With that in mind, let me try again. Can we see trigger tapes from that time as the website, blogs, Instastories, and Snapchats of today, interactive media intended to spark conversation and share information?

ALEX: Again, yes and no. Yes, in the sense that a group of people were engaged in making and sharing media to draw awareness and support for their own communities. But no, in the sense that in the 1980s and 90s, pre-internet, these mediated encounters were more conversational and communal at every step along the way than digital media feels today (even as more users generate it, and even interact through hashtags, forwarding, liking, and commenting). People make websites by themselves all the time, and of course people access information on websites by themselves all the time. But these trigger tapes, and a good deal of early AIDS activist video, were not individual undertakings. Maybe they were closer to something like a website plus a meetup group, but even that does not capture the ideological and practical foundation of collaboration and on-the-ground education and movement-making that was at the heart of many of the tapes that I cared most deeply about at the time, and which I have to say also formed the core of my own AIDS activist video response.

 This is a technological, political, representational condition of AIDS Crisis Culture: it was social, interactive, shared. In this sense, it was the *mak-*

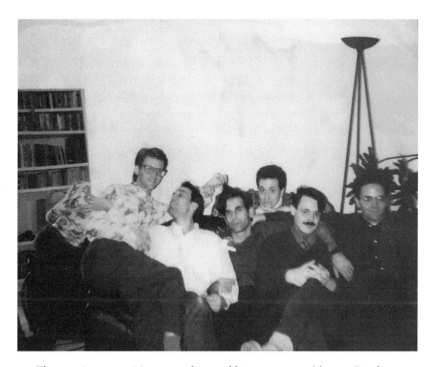

4.1 The consciousness-raising group that would go on to create Silence = Death. From left to right: Avram Finkelstein, Charles Kreloff, Jorge Socarrás, Brian Howard, Chris Lione, Oliver Johnston. Photo courtesy of Avram Finkelstein.

ing of the trigger tapes (and most other AIDS activist videos in the earlier period) that comes closest to a consciousness-raising group. The studying, encounters, and politicizing necessary to make video resulted in a material output with social change goals rather than primarily an internal and personal change or the quick but untraceable sharing of things through digital culture and its glut of private aha moments that infuse our current relations with images and ideas on the internet. With digital culture, each interaction is exciting, but also interchangeable and somehow hard to hold on to, given the guarantee that another will so quickly follow. Political, educational, and artistic impact are almost entirely privatized in production and reception today, to be linked technologically, yes, but so as to create an immediate but harder-to-sustain power and buzz.

TED: Right, so the idea of people together in time and space is really important. And it reminds me of Dirty Looks, the film screening series that was

69

started in 2012 by Bradford Nordeen and friends. Early Dirty Looks collaborator and staffer Karl McCool once gave me some background on their goals: "When Dirty Looks started we were inspired by this idea of film societies and cinema clubs in the 60s in the New York Underground, this idea that artists and cinephiles and the general public would come together in a social space and experience experimental film, not as a museum piece but as part of community."[4] Which then makes me also think of theorists Stefano Harney and Fred Moten's definition of "study," which Moten shares in an interview with Stephen Shukaitis: "I think we were committed to the idea that study is what you do with other people. It's talking and walking around with other people, working, dancing, suffering, some irreducible convergence of all three, held under the name of speculative practice."[5] That seems closer to what you are getting at.

ALEX: That's really useful, Ted. And that is what I mean! At that time, more so than it seems now, AIDS (and much else) was lived as a collective experience, so yes, in the working, dancing, and suffering of our lives together we were "studying." We had no choice. Before the meds came out in 1996 (which was a decade after the HIV antibody test came out and fifteen years after HIV was first "discovered"), we not only lived with HIV together, but we also responded together in self-made, sometimes interlocking corners of a larger world of AIDS, and also its representations. Because there was less total representation (about anything), because video was harder to make and show than it is now (although much easier than making film, the reason why so many of us gravitated to the format at the moment when consumer cameras and editing first became available), because distribution wasn't as easy to facilitate and so tapes were not so readily accessible, people mostly watched things together on screens, and our videos were often held in carefully curated collections to be made available to others who needed them. We made and watched video communally and in conversation with our allies and friends, our larger if still specific intended audiences, and those viewers who got to them in their own, unanticipated ways.

With the three vignettes on the Bebashi tape, the quality of the tape pales in comparison to the caliber of interaction that it reveals and can also stimulate. This was a pretty common set of goals: to make something that we were proud of, that we could show to each other, and that would be of use. And the making of the video was where a good deal of where the world-changing was taking place: naming things, choosing what to highlight and share, hashing out analyses and stories together, being willing to self-represent in a time when this was rarely done for any regular person on their own terms or by themselves, let alone for disenfranchised people like women of color, poor people, drug users, abused women, Black women in Philadelphia, or people ill and dying: the communities always at the heart of AIDS stories of tragedy, trauma, connection, and empowerment.

TED: I think I speak for both of us when I say we see our work here as a *trigger book*! A trigger tape gives us difficult prompts, not to figure something out finally, but to stop and ideally think about in proximity, out loud, and together. Better yet, tape allows us something harder and perhaps even more important: a fixed record that can help and prompt us to think about how processes and issues also change in time.

TRIGGER 4
BEING
TRIGGERED
IN TIMES

1 **READ**

"Teaching Tolerance," a free guide to have conversations around race and racism, http://www.tolerance.org/sites/default/files/general /TT%20Difficult%20Conversations%20web.pdf.

2 **CONSIDER**

Two readings about teaching with triggers:

- 7 Humanities Professors. "Trigger Warnings Are Flawed." *Inside Higher Ed*, May 29, 2014. https://www.insidehighered.com/views /2014/05/29/essay-faculty-members-about-why-they-will-not-use -trigger-warnings.
- Angela Carter. "Teaching with Trauma: Trigger Warnings, Feminism, and Disability Pedagogy." *Disability Studies Quarterly* 35, no. 2 (Spring 2015). https://dsq-sds.org/article/view/4652/3935.

3 **REWATCH**

Pause the Bebashi tape at one of the three fades to black. Consider the sequence left in medias res. If you were in that situation, what would you do?

TRIGGER 5
BEING TRIGGERED BY ABSENCE

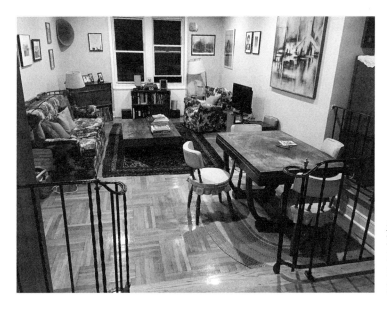

5.1 Alex's living room in Ditmas Park, Brooklyn. Nighttime.

TED: I was a bit tired the first time I watched the Bebashi tape. It was 2016, it was late evening, and we were in your living room. We were actually watching a bunch of your tapes in anticipation of a conference where we would be presenting AIDS video from the past to illustrate understandings of HIV/AIDS that have not been dragged forward over time. Maybe we had dinner first? I am sure I brought over sparkling water, maybe chocolate. And maybe this was the first time we watched something together at the same time in the same place.

ALEX: Yes. My crappy DVD player didn't work and you had to go home to get yours.

TED: Is that true? I remember your broken DVD player but I think in the end you got it to work.

ALEX: I actually had to buy a new one. The cheapest one on Amazon.

TED: I do remember it was summer. And if I can be frank, I remember being surprised that you did not have a bigger screen.

ALEX: If that's the biggest surprise about how I live my life that you have encountered now that we really know each other then I feel pretty well seen! And not to be too didactic or pedantic here, but a lot of our work is about seeing beyond simple assumptions based upon what at first look seems like obvious clues (rooted in race or class or age, say), as well as about learning how to look when there are no clues to be found.

For example, we don't know the year that the tape was made, and even our attempts to fact-check with Bebashi staff have not turned up conclusive results. But we can make some guesses. Bebashi did not open until 1985, and I defended my dissertation in 1991. I would have most likely already watched the vignettes by then, although I did return to New York from Philadelphia (where I was teaching from 1991 to 1995) to do more research and writing while I was transforming my dissertation into a monograph for publication.

TED: So we are guessing that the tape is late 1980s, and maybe as late as 1990. But most likely not 1991.

ALEX: Exactly. Which is interesting to me because I remember much of the early to mid-1990s so well. 1994 was the year after my best friend Jim died of AIDS. I was in New York City to grieve and heal and remember. I watched a lot of tapes at that time and my work and life was something like an AIDS cocoon. I was subletting a small studio on East 10th Street surrounded by images of AIDS and underlined by the loss of a man with whom I had first come to New York, and into my adulthood, and for whom I continue to do my AIDS-related memory work and ongoing activism.

TED: His loss allowed for other things to be saved. Early in our research, I contacted Bebashi by email to try to find out more about "Grandma's Legacy." I was told that information about the video production *was* available. It could be found, they wrote to me . . . wait for it . . . in a book. In your book! It was a closed loop that led us back to you. To me, this suggests how much was happening, and maybe how fast it was all being produced.

ALEX: Well, if you are suggesting that things were happening so fast during AIDS Crisis Culture that proper records were not being kept, I would say that would be true for the underfunded agencies doing a lot of the work. If you are noticing that cultural and even institutional history stays vivid only across micro-generations: yes again. And if you are noting how small, self-referential, and self-dependent was the AIDS activist culture of the early years (as it is now), this is critical. But also, I wrote about this tape then, because as is true now, I think local, community-made video is of critical importance even if, and sort of because it receives little to no official or mainstream cultural sanction (and not that much from scholars, either, I have to admit): in terms of funding, being seen, being saved, being written about, or rewatched. What needs more love than hardly touched and little-seen objects?! And activist video works so well because it does what mainstream media never can: be precise, local, difficult, honest, opinionated, offensive, inscrutable, messy, and sincere.

To be honest, I'm not sure how many other people in the world care about this video or even this *type* of video. I hope our writing models why one might . . . But I also know that the numbers of viewers, or carers even, can never be a rubric that will work for understanding the kinds of AIDS activism that I care about.

TED: Right. It is about connections.

ALEX: Not counts. I, too, made *We Care: A Video for Care Providers of People Affected by AIDS* (1990) in a video collective made primarily of women of color (the Women's AIDS Video Enterprise, WAVE) and in a sister community (Brooklyn, New York) and AIDS Service Organization (ASO), the Brooklyn AIDS Task Force, and with a complementary method (collectively produced media by for our own community). As much as we were angry and passionate and fast, we took what we were doing very seriously. People's lives depended on a careful relay of the information we were attempting to disseminate. People were hungry for honest reflections of their own experiences. And given that videomaking was hard, the equipment was only starting to become available, and none of us exactly felt authorized to speak, we bolstered each other into making visible aspects of our own lives that hadn't been much seen (as moving image media).

75

TED: So you were making visible something that hadn't been seen? Why, or perhaps better yet, for whom?

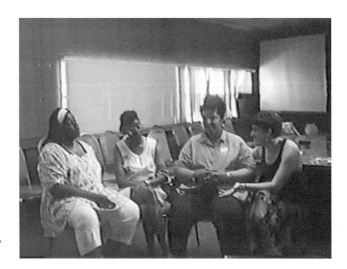

5.2 Screen grab, *We Care: A Video for Care Providers of People Affected by* AIDS (WAVE, 1990).

ALEX: We knew we were accountable to people in our communities or movements or homes. But we were present-focused. So this meant that maybe we weren't all that thoughtful about being accountable to unimaginable people in the future (like us, now, Ted, hoping for records). Rather, we were there for each other. And we were there for the people we knew who could not be present (on camera) because of access and privilege, illness, time, or self-confidence. Many of us were barely adults and yet we were trying to save each other and others. We had to be brazen and empowered because people around us were sick and dying. Some of us got grants from city and state governmental agencies, or from arts organizations and nonprofits (for instance, my $25,000 from the New York State Council for the Humanities, awarded with a lot of help, I must admit, from program officer Coco Fusco, who went on to be an important artist and critic in her own right). Some of us didn't get any grants and made our work for nothing. There are records of how we interacted with institutions. I still have file after file of the grants applications that I was awarded or mostly denied. They are also in my office, as dusty and dated in format as the VHS tapes we're now digitizing (the majority of these files were paper-based documents, typed or handwritten, and this not on computers!). My files hold fliers for screenings that we pasted on walls, and handwritten notes we mailed to each other in thanks. And lists! I have a lot of lists of tapes that maybe I watched, or maybe were just possible to watch, if I went to the AIDS Library of Philadelphia, for instance.

TED: What do you mean, lists?

76

AIDS LIBRARY of Phila.

VIDEO COLLECTION

Title	# Copies
Special report on AIDS (1985)	c.1, 2
AIDS / Sally Jesse Raphael Show (1987)	c.1
AIDS special (1987)	c.1
The AIDS quarterly: spring 1989	c.1, 2, 3
The AIDS quarterly: winter 1989	c.2
The AIDS quarterly: 2/89; AIDS now (1-4)	c.1
AIDS now (5, 6); the AIDS quarterly: 4/89; 1, 11/90;	
AIDS in rural America	c.1
The AIDS quarterly: winter 1990	c.1, 2
Longtime companions (1990)	c.1, 2
Phila. AIDS Task Force	
An introduction for volunteers	c.1
How to avoid burnout (Shanti, 9)	c.1, 2
Condom talk	c.1
Introduction to grief (Shanti, 14)	c.1, 2
Not a silent dying (1991)	c.1
PWA support group (1; Shanti, 19)	c.2
The new tradition: safer sex counseling ...	c.1

5.3 A list of AIDS tapes from Alex's files.

ALEX: When I was going through my files to prepare for our conversation I found folders of paper-based stuff, including a list of tapes which I think might have been held by Bebashi! It is a good reminder that "Grandma's Legacy" was just one of many projects created in a short amount of time by diverse and fledgling artists. Think about the output coming out of just one ASO in Philly, and then think about the cultural production at all the ASOs across the country and then the world. What this means decades later is that I can come across a list of tapes and not really recognize any of them (the tapes or the list) in any useful way. And even though this list was recorded and saved, most of the details of our efforts, and productions, and our conversations that made them happen went *unrecorded* (they were less important than getting the tape made and sent out), or they were recorded and then shredded when someone left a job: "That video was a very long time ago." All of which is to say, I think the lack of available records in the present tells us very little about the work we were doing in the past and instead more about the afterlife of attention, care, and priorities as the crisis has worn on.

TED: So: enter the idea that something not being present matters. Absence can be a clue, a path to understanding. A lack tells us something. My guess would be as the epidemic continued throughout the 1990s and into the twenty-first century, well after the introduction of life-saving medication became accessible in 1996—when attention and funding veered in new directions and the Second Silence began—the overworked and underpaid employees of this AIDS nonprofit, like those all over the world, some of which I have worked at, did not know what to make of their collection of VHS tapes and affiliated records and so they put them somewhere deep in the organization's storage. Or because of space or other pressing issues, they decided to get rid of the tapes altogether, overwhelmed as we all are by the costs, demands, and upkeep of new technology as well as the ever present and changing concerns of HIV/AIDS.

ALEX: People stopped using VHS as they bought new cameras and decks. I had to re-render all my work as DVDs only to then digitize them.

TED: It's funny, right? Shifts in technology mean we can lose access to information we thought we had. Information that was ours to begin with, and hard won at that! But I think as we engage the Bebashi tape here, from a variety of approaches, something is gained, even in loss, when we find something else, more than information really, something like an essence.

ALEX: Can you say more?

TED: I am thinking of *Listening to Images* by Tina Campt, in which she suggests that sound is an important aspect of engaging with institutional photos of Black people.[1] In thinking about our project watching the Bebashi tape, I find Campt's ideas helpful, specifically her thinking around how a scarcity of images is not always a lack, per se. She is inviting us to think very profoundly about listening. And this is beyond what a human ear may or may not be able to do. It is about the senses. For example, within an absence of images that might explicitly represent what we are looking for—say, representations of Black people, or women, or trans folks within the AIDS archive—there is an invitation to us to consider how what we are looking for might be or is actually already present, albeit through sound, vibrations, frequency, and so on. And I would add is also made present by our questions, our yearning, and our awareness/hope for connection.

ALEX: I hear you (ha), but I don't want to lose the fact that for some people that might not be good enough. They want materials, be that as proof or so that what they yearn for can be reproducible and thus shareable. This gets us back to the importance of the object as a platform for process: memory, community, pride, history, conversation. In a lot of ways this is what the Fae Richards Archive (Zoe Leonard and Cheryl Dunye) and our film that uses it, *The Watermelon Woman* (Dunye, 1996) does and is also about. It falsifies the objects that Black lesbians most need and understands the truth in this desire for evidence, even if it is "fake."

TED: Right, so a challenge becomes how to bring sense to that which is not visibly obvious but truthfully felt. Key to Campt's book is the power of refusal and what that makes undeniable. Having something physical, something you can point to, like the function of the (fake but so very real) Fae Richards archive of eighty-two photos, is an example. The invitation to listen to the archives for the vibrations of what is not visible or immediate is related to the act of refusal, an "extension of the range of creative responses Black communities have marshalled in the face of racialized dispossession."[2] For me Campt is saying that a person not being hyper-visible, or rather being thoughtful in how they are visible, is a survival tactic that is explicitly about futurity and its hopeful radical project of being found, later. Being sensed in the archive has less to do with just being and is more about being found by someone who is searching with subtly, dignity, and respect from and for the margins (sonic, visual, social, and otherwise).

What does it mean to listen to activist AIDS video from AIDS Crisis Culture, in both a practical but also maybe deeper sense? How can our conversational method disrupt and open up archival practices beyond looking for or even finding what is immediately visible? How do we respect and honor all of our senses, including sound, while respecting that not everything "lost" needs to be found?

ALEX: The past presents itself to you not as you wish it was, but as it might be, and that can be transformative; like me not having a big TV, or any other fancy gizmos in my apartment for that matter. I'm some mix of cheap and funky and snobbish, I suppose.

TED: Ha! Yeah, exactly. Going to your house to watch the videos helped me see that we don't always get what we want: like a new film professor neighbor with a kick-ass home entertainment system where I could invite myself over to watch *Grace and Frankie* when not watching AIDS tapes.

But seriously, maybe after reading our effort here, another of those Bebashi volunteers or staff members will contact us and we will gain even more insight into the history of this tape: what drove her, or people like her, to this particular instance of self-representation and community-based care. Our project is about generating dynamism about and from the past and ongoing experiences of HIV/AIDS through objects, and the people who make, use, and need them.

ALEX: Or maybe they won't ever call us with more info. And that is okay as well. As much as we have made meaning out of this tape that helps us now, maybe for the people involved, it does not carry the same investment. Maybe it was one of thirty projects they did that year, or they don't really remember doing it.

TED: Or they don't want to think back about that day, that time in their lives. There was a moment when Abdul-Khabeer was thinking about how she might be able to track down the women who worked on the tape, and she just kind of trailed off mid-sentence.

ALEX: And you didn't follow up?

TED: No. Because I trusted whatever process she was going through. At the end of the day, she has a history with the tape's makers and the tape that we don't. I can only assume she was weighing the possibilities and impacts of remaking connections. And in the end, in that moment, she paused.

ALEX: I get it. Over the long history of the WAVE collective, many of us have disappeared ourselves from ongoing conversation about the tape, for any number of reasons—including how painful it is given that some of the people we were caring for then died a long time ago, or for religious reasons—while some of us still get together to catch up. And that is okay.

TED: When it comes to AIDS, we have learned that even amid the pain of loss, absence can be generative, and finding things can be beautiful. I guess leaving things behind can have its own range of emotions. We're certainly not celebrating loss, just saying we can make use of it. But saving is good, too!

ALEX: The Bebashi tape survives for us to engage with because I have always valued community-based AIDS video. And I never moved on entirely. I have been lucky enough to have had steady employment, and an office where I can safely store things like tapes. As a professor moving up the ranks, I have been able to maintain my activist, academic, and creative practice within the AIDS Response over many decades, dragging along with me my personal and institutional memories and many of the things that document these. I've worked through many of my memories and documents, even as I've allowed others to slumber. Bebashi may not have that exact luxury of a stable place or time to save their VHS tapes because they had and have other things to do that are even more critical.

TED: Last year I met with Gary J. Bell, the current executive director of Bebashi, to talk about the tape. As you know, there is not really any institutional memory about it. Nevertheless, the input, needs, and centering of Black women living with HIV remain key to the organization.

ALEX: What seems clear in these discussions with Abdul-Khabeer and Bell is that the tape was one minor but not inconsequential manifestation of their ethics and process over years of AIDS work.

TED: So we could argue that as long as the commitments are being dragged forward in time, the tape is not as important as the work they are doing.

ALEX: What it also makes clear is that our inability to find records is just one part of the story. I kept their tape, and wrote a book about other things like it decades ago. A multifaceted network of archivists and historians, activists, professors, and social workers, all in conversation with each other, can allow for a richer grasp of what we once knew, didn't or don't know, what we have learned and know now, and what we might still figure out together.

TED: I feel that the best responses to HIV/AIDS mirror experiences of the epidemic. There should be intimacy, it should be transmittable in some way, and I think what you are getting at: all this should be interactive.

TRIGGER 5
BEING TRIGGERED
BY ABSENCE

1 **MIRROR AN EXPERIENCE OF THE EPIDEMIC**

Talk again about the vignette that you were triggered by when answering Trigger 4, this time by looking for its gaps, silences, and what is left unsaid or undone.

2 **LISTEN**

Three resources that ask us to listen about women, AIDS, and race. What do you hear? What stays absent but true?

- The ACT UP Oral History Project. Accessed November 14, 2021. http://www.actuporalhistory.org.
- Jennifer Brier and Matthew Wizinsky. "'I'm Still Surviving': A Women's History of HIV." Oral history project, Women of the Chicago Women's Interagency HIV Study. Humanities for All. Accessed November 14, 2021. https://humanitiesforall.org/projects /im-still-surviving.
- Alyson Campbell. "GL RY: A (W)hole lot of Woman Trouble: HIV Dramaturgies and Feral Pedagogies." In *Viral Dramaturgies: HIV and AIDS in Performance in the Twenty-First Century*, edited by Alyson Campbell and Dirk Gindt, 49–67. London: Palgrave Macmillan, 2018.

TRIGGER 6

HOW TO HAVE AN AIDS MEMORIAL IN AN EPIDEMIC

TED: I was really moved when the grandma says, "You know how it is when people die? Folks always be putting words in your mouth. This way, if I don't say it on tape, I ain't say it, baby." For me this indexes this tape as the form of memorial in which I'm most interested: an activist, participatory version in which the person who will be dying plays a role in how they will be remembered.

ALEX: It is right there in the name: "Grandma's Legacy." The mother and daughter are working together to build a bridge between the grandma and the unborn grandchild, aware that, due to the impact of the virus and the nonavailability of medical support at the time, the grandmother will not live long enough to be witnessed or known by her daughter's child.

TED: And for me, if we understand that the tape is actually for the local community (with the granddaughter as a stand-in), we see its political aspect as well. It is also about collecting the experiences, voices, and lived realities of Black women living with HIV. Stories like this would be known to those in the local community—maybe—but they were unrepresented elsewhere.

ALEX: In *We Care*, some members of the WAVE collective visit the home of Marie, an African American grandmother living with HIV. We made that tape in 1990, and she was closeted about her HIV status because of the extreme stigma, and related violence, that was total and definitive at this time. It was one of only a tiny number of such images of a Black woman with AIDS from this period that I am aware of. Fictionalizing the story in the Bebashi tape is one important form of protection, but I also want to note that real stories and lives like this were also hidden from the local community. So making them visible was fully political, as Marie understood for our tape.

TED: Marie is so powerful, as is the footage you shot of her. You, Juanita, and I, along with others, have shown that tape a lot in recent years, and it resonates with a kind of power I think must have been present back in the day.

ALEX: Yes and no. A few years ago I showed it in LA, and over post-screening grub, another panelist wanted to talk about the footage as "poverty porn." If you remember, I was so taken aback by this comment that I called you right after.

TED: Yeah, I was as shocked as you were. It seemed to me that he was either projecting or was unaware of New York apartments.

ALEX: Exactly. Marie's place is the epitome of working or even middle-class New York! She has a decent-sized one-bedroom. There is nothing poor about the scene outside of the VHS tape we shot it on. And even if she did live in poverty, that can be made visible and not be an aspect of a contemporary consumptive intrusive viewing practice. Some people living with HIV do live in poverty, and in fact that should be seen as well, if for no other reason than that it is true and important. In this case it was Sharon, her partner and a member of WAVE, and I who shot Marie's tour of her apartment.

The point of taping the visit with Marie was to illustrate the everydayness of a Black woman living with HIV who is an integral part of her community and family. The fact that she happens to have a well-furnished, tidy one bedroom is beside the point, but information nonetheless.

TED: The comment about poverty also suggested that there was a lack of appreciation of Marie's agency in the project, and so maybe a misunderstanding of the politics of the work.

84   ALEX: There is a conflation of race, class, and nonagency. Like, because someone is Black and working-class we can't see them outside of current patterns

of spectacle and humiliation. In its moment, the tape was understood by viewers to depict openness and invitation as well as a kind of media-enabled authority. Because it was primarily shown peer to peer (with the occasional art gallery or community theater screening) there was a shared awareness of what was being seen and shown, as well as by and for whom. Maybe my fellow panelist who worried about poverty porn has been too inundated by manipulative reality TV to understand that someone in front of the camera can be an active participant in cocreation. Representing poverty in and of itself does not equal the objectifying pleasures derived from porn.

TED: Which brings us back to the Bebashi tape. Would it also be seen as poverty porn? Poverty of ASO resources? Or can people appreciate it for what it is: people and networks stretching themselves beyond capacity to care for and save each other though media? Like *We Care*, we can understand Bebashi's tape as one from an outpouring of AIDS cultural production from the early years of the epidemic that provide voice, inclusion, direction, and representation to the quickly developing media ecology around AIDS. Twenty-first-century AIDS activism is about safeguarding all that was fought for over the years—like a comprehensive agenda about drugs, housing, and poverty or decreasing stigma, discrimination, and criminalization—while also tending to the ongoing ramifications of the war on drugs, as well as racism, poverty, transphobia, misogyny, homophobia, etc. And as was true for the past, the most helpful and insightful communication of this comes from the people most impacted, those carrying the heaviest burdens of the crisis, and shouldering the bulk of the resistance. Specifically here I am thinking about the HIV/ Prison Abolitionist/ Fair Housing activist group, VOCAL, who understand and state that we could end the crisis tomorrow without a cure, if we tended to the needs of people living with HIV who are made the most marginalized.[1]

ALEX: I love how this example links contemporary politics to earlier efforts. For the Bebashi tape, a community AIDS organization mustered their resources— community members, analyses, the money they needed to rent or buy equipment—to break into representation and stop the erasure of Black women by representing this for themselves. Do you think the Bebashi tape creates a memorial, via fiction, for one grandma with HIV on a tape, a memorial for Black women of a certain age who died of AIDS, otherwise too often forgotten, neglected, or written out of the history of the seen?

TED: I agree with your use of the word "fiction," as it is a memorial for a character who stands in for real people. Beyond that I would say I am invested in thinking with you about what it means for these two women to make this document together—whether it is a memorial or not—while the grandma is still living. That is powerful, to use tape for self-representation in the face of death.

ALEX: That is one of the reasons camcorders seemed so revolutionizing to us in the 1980s, when they first became available. They allowed consumers, regular people, access to the discrete evidentiary powers of moving image-making: "If I don't say it on tape." While video is made for people and movements in its moment, it is always also for the future because it is built to capture and save. This video was also made for us who are alive now.

TED: For sure. But I think something inherent in our work is this question: How and why do you memorialize something while it is still ongoing?

ALEX: This is central to our exploration of video as method and medium and metaphor (for generation loss and recovery). Video is a technology engaged in and with a lived present, but it also has the capacity and intention of being engaged again and again in the future. Something we can't exactly know because we don't know the women involved in the making of the Bebashi tape is what they imagined the future to be. We know they were making the tape for "the granddaughter," someone who would be aware of AIDS because her grandmother lived with it and was willing to be recorded testifying to this truth as she was dying.

TED: Maybe they were able to imagine the very present we are in, where there are now as many if not more people living worldwide with HIV than have ever died with the virus. Maybe, because of their lived experience, they knew that the future would be a world where AIDS was still an epidemic but one largely forgotten by the general public because it was and is still impacting, damaging, and killing people from marginalized communities such as gay men, trans women, Black people, queer men of color, poor people, etc.

ALEX: Using the grandmother's words in the Bebashi video as one of our guides, we need to ask what it means when recorded words meant to represent those living with HIV and those deeply impacted, so as to save and then move them into the future, are secured only then again to become lost. What does an AIDS activist media archive, and its congruent history look like, if it is seen through the eyes of Black women and the organizations that served and serve them and which they often run/ran? And how can we learn from this as white people? HIV-negative people? People from different classes or local backgrounds?

86

TED: Throughout this conversation, a song keeps coming to mind: Erykah Badu's "A.D. 2000," in which she sings, "You won't be naming no buildings after me. To go down dilapidated. My name mis-stated." For me, this song lends itself to memorials in the two ways we are talking about: the literal (if fictional) way a person can be remembered (Ms. Bennett), but also the collective way that a group of people (be it Black women, people with AIDS, Black women with AIDS) become part of the future. For Badu, a built structure is not the way to go; it falls apart, and for all intents and purposes does not carry forward the soul of the person: "My name mis-stated." I played this song for my students in a class I was teaching about how to memorialize AIDS while it is ongoing, and the song conjured up a discussion of the Shirley Chisholm building in downtown Brooklyn. My students had not noticed the name of the building, and even if they had, it did not really inspire more connections because they did not know who Chisholm was. And no name on a building—mis-stated or otherwise—is going to easily correct that.

ALEX: Did you tell them who she was? That she was a politician, and in 1972 was the first Black woman to run for president with the fierce campaign slogan, "Unbossed and Unbothered"?

TED: I did. And I asked them what could the building do to actually honor or even conjure Ms. Chisholm? We bandied about the possibility of a small exhibition in the lobby, or an app that would provide some history to those inquisitive enough to take a look. But in the end, the best idea was a simple one: including an image of Chisholm on the side of the building. The reasoning being, we still live in a political moment where having a building named after a Black woman is noteworthy. That is to say, we still think there is a social gain to be made in honoring a prominent Black woman, publicly, because she is worthy of being celebrated, and because systemic bias burdens Black women and decreases their life chances. Naming a building after Chisholm is an example of memorializing something while it is still an ongoing concern, issue, and reality. And so the takeaway for me was: broadly speaking, naming something is not enough. There is no actual legacy work being done that can't and won't be easily ignored, disrespected, or eradicated over time. And I think that is what Badu is saying as well.

ALEX: To me the song is about controlling all aspects of the representational cycle, a way of thinking about media power that is rather antithetical to today's culture where the amount of attention, via hits or views, is the primary metric we use to prove how successful is any image. This is to say, we live in

87

a time where a small but growing number of Black women are more visible, or even hyper-visible, but are they controlling how these images circulate, where they land, what gets done with them and by whom, how their names are spoken and with what feeling? And what about the rest of us who never have large numbers of people who see us or want to hear what we tweet or shoot? I'd much rather stay small and local and thus be able to experience and verify that there is an accuracy of intention, audience, and understanding to my legacy.

TED: That makes sense, and I think this is similar to the strategy being employed by the fictional mother and daughter in "Grandma's Legacy," and the very nonfictional if still unknown people who created, wrote, and shot it.

ALEX: Ted, as you know, the makers of the Bebashi tape are from a similar generation as me, a generation that for better or worse got very good at marking death as an emotional, cultural, and political aspect of AIDS (Debra Levine's work on AIDS political funerals is noteworthy).[2] Within the same decade when "Grandma's Legacy" was made, we also have the Mary's from ACT UP who were inspired by David Wojnarowicz and began producing political funerals.[3] We understood that death was a moment of both remembrance and media, and that while it was about mourning, it was also an opportunity for organizing.

Amid all the death and governmental neglect (and yes, hope, sex, and youth) there was (and remains) a constant need to remind "the outside world" that AIDS is not over. The first version of this slogan was a 1986 sticker by Little Elvis. Please, for me, imagine what the climate must have been like that an artist collective felt the need to remind people that a violent plague unrolling all over the world was "not over." Imagine the erasure, isolation, general public apathy, and media blackout that was occurring even as we were seeing our friends, neighborhoods, and communities decimated, even as you and I call this period AIDS Crisis Culture, to indicate its scope, volume, and saturation.

TED: Thank you for saying that, and I think that that same confluence of anxiety, death, sadness, and open questions about the future is very much still at play when we talk now about how to have memorials within an epidemic. I think there is real stress today that not only has the past been forgotten, but the present is being overlooked.

ALEX: And there's that contradiction, first expressed so powerfully by Douglas Crimp in "Mourning and Militancy."[4] For both activists and PWAs, should we be remembering instead of seeing or fighting?

THE AIDS CRISIS IS NOT OVER

6.1 Little Elvis, The AIDS Crisis Is Not Over sticker, 1988.

TED: The fears raised about a forgotten present is only increasing in the face of a resurgence of interest in the past of AIDS (AIDS Crisis Revisitation), as seen through the recent and voluminous release of movies, books, and art exhibitions about early responses to AIDS. On top of, or as part of this, there is a recent wave of AIDS memorials such as the one in New York City that opened up in 2016, and the one slated for completion in 2023–24 in LA. Amid all this remembering, there is so much forgetting or not seeing what is right there: specifically, Black people, Black women, and the influence they have had and do have on the AIDS Response, and the impact of the virus on Black women, men, femmes, queers, trans, and other people from marginalized communities.

ALEX: Yes, and as "Grandma's Legacy" testifies, that very real and profound analysis and anxiety is neither new, nor unfounded.

TED: So the question is, how do memorials even begin to hold space for all that they need to contain? To begin to consider these questions and ideas, I worked with my previously mentioned class to come up with some significant aspects of what an AIDS memorial needs to include to be meaningful and helpful in multiple capacities:

1. Maintain and build upon the activist goals of the movement.
2. Create culture about the past, present, and future of AIDS.
3. Say not only the names of people who died with HIV, but also share the ways they lived, the tactics they used to love, fight, die, etc.
4. Reflect aspects of the crisis itself: collaborative, intimate, and involving risk, and being replicable and also disruptive, educational, and changeable over time, thereby accumulating meaning, stories, and history.

89

ALEX: I'm very impressed by this list, Ted, and the work you did with your students over the course of a semester. That leaves me feeling encouraged. With attention, focus, and interest, the political, personal, and artistic complexities of the history and present of AIDS are available to people who are intimate with, or only interested in, the ongoing crisis. Did your students think things like the Bebashi tape were *memorials*? It seems to sit firmly grounded in the rubric above.

TED: As part of the class we spoke about memorials, like the one in New York, but for us, more importantly, we began to discuss countermemorials, an idea that I have come to understand through the work of James Young.[5] He talks about how a successful memorial does not allow the object to do the heavy lifting of remembering. This is a problematic offloading of the human task of memory work. He says good countermemorials index the past and place the memory work back on individuals and communities. This is something we are thinking through here when it comes to cultural production. I see "Grandma's Legacy," a trigger tape made for public interactive consumption and discussion, as an example of a countermemorial. I think the format of the tape demands audience lifting.

ALEX: I really like this. It aligns with some of my own earlier writing about AIDS memorials (online), where the ease of consumption (and in some cases production) minimize the fact that grieving, remembering, and memorializing should all be *hard*.[6] Memorials matter for me if the dead are honored as would make them feel seen, but also in ways that help us to feel seen now; when their messages are heard in ways where their words instigate new connections so that visitors are touched into action. We need each other, we need amplification of less heard voices, and we need better circulation of things that would otherwise be lost to history.

TED: What has to be in place for media to be a helpful form of archive and memorial?

ALEX: In my work on the VHS Archives project—another place where I have been thinking about the legacy of my collection of tapes with you and others— it is our assertion that things and their formats are not really that important (building, tape, song), what matters most is if they can be used in ways that connect to people with needs in the present. So what is most significant is a hungry, agile, engaged audience (as small as is necessary) in the present, to activate and use an archive well. The more local the better, not really in the meaning of lived place or shared identity, but in a knowingness to the other or others involved in the looking and a knowingness about the thing and what they might want to do with it.

TED: Yeah, agreed. Form matters only as a guide. And this becomes interesting when you expand Young's notion of countermemorial. For him, a memorial is not just the thing that gets built, or even the thing that does not get built, but also the stories around the process. He comes from Holocaust studies, and for him, the discussions that center around the hows and whys that go into understanding what needs to be created are part of the memorial process. Similarly, Emilie Townes's idea of countermemories, from her 2006 *Womanist Ethics and the Cultural Production of Evil*, raises the idea that naming the incompleteness of most histories that fail to include Black women and Black lives is not enough. She is interested and invested in looking to the past for microhistories—the stories of individual Black women and their relations— as a way to refocus enshrined narratives. She writes, "Countermemory can open up subversive spaces within dominant discourse that expand our sense of who we are and, possibly, create a more whole and just society in defiance of structural evil."[7] Memorial then is not just how we remember; we must also consider how we as cultures unremember, and thereby make space for countermemory and microhistories.

ALEX: Along those lines I think Dagmawi Woubshet's work is really critical. In his book *The Calendar of Loss*, he traces notions of grief and ritual that are live now while connecting to patterns of mourning that came out of the AIDS crisis in the 1980s and 1990s in Ethiopia.[8] He, as it seems we are suggesting here, also puts forward an idea of memorial as process, one that is live and includes the past. Similarly, Ira Sachs's tape *Last Address* (2010) remembers gay men from New York City's East Village who died of AIDS, and the apartments they lived in that stand there still. But it may be the yearly tours of these very still sites, created by Alex Fialho for Visual AIDS, that are the memorials that can move and change us now.[9]

Building upon that, I think that a memorial can be remembering in any form—built or not built, still or moving—and its sources are not big H history, but the stories we tell, and the stories that don't get told, the lives lived, our memories, and some reclaimed tapes.

TED: I think so, and I think our work outside of this conversation and including our discussions of "Grandma's Legacy" is part of counterhistories and countermemorialization.

91

ALEX: So is our conversation here an activity of memorial? Or a form of memorialization?

TED: What do you think?

ALEX: I think we need not only have access to the things we made, but also to own our own carefully developed and refined processes of reengagement in order to bring forward the past of AIDS into the present. Be that from thirty years ago, or yesterday. So yes, if I am understanding Young, Townes, and you correctly, conversation, as it relates to AIDS video, can be a useful form of memorialization within an epidemic if done with shared purpose for the present. And I think "Grandma's Legacy" on its own is a memorial, and—maybe most interestingly for me, in thinking about your guidelines for what makes an effective AIDS memorial—so is our conversation, and then also our invitation to readers to consider the tape: these are both forms of meaningful countermemory and memorialization.

TED: We can relate this back to Badu's song. I think she is singing an idea that Young is writing about. A building or a built monument can never do what our hearts and minds working together and collectively are capable of. Our most meaningful connection to the past is our memories. Objects—like a video tape—can take us close, but they cannot replace memory, which is internal and personal and expansive.

ALEX: Are you saying that a memorial can be a trigger? It creates a public through its audience and then invites them to consider, engage, and perhaps begin to change together. So "Grandma's Legacy" is a memorial in content and form. And then memorial, if we are following the lead of "Grandma's Legacy" and the Bebashi tape as a whole, this is about memorializing alongside living, and this is one approach to having an AIDS memorial in an epidemic.

TRIGGER 6
HOW TO
HAVE AN AIDS
MEMORIAL IN
AN EPIDEMIC

1 **VISIT**

AIDSMemorial.info and AIDSMemorial.org//interactive-aids-quilt.

2 **READ**
 - Marita Sturken. *Tangled Memories: The Vietnam War, the AIDS Epi-demic, and the Politics of Remembering.* Berkeley: University of California Press, 1997.
 - Emilie Townes. *Womanist Ethics and the Cultural Production of Evil.* London: Palgrave Macmillan, 2006.
 - James Young. *The Stages of Memory: Reflections on Memorial Art, Loss, and the Spaces Between.* Amherst: University of Massachusetts Press, 2016.

3 **FIND**

Are histories of AIDS represented publicly where you live? How, where, by and for whom? If not, listen to this absence.

AN AIDS CONVERSATION SCRIPT TO BE READ ALOUD
TIMELINE 2

Use this script with a group, one other person, or by yourself. Ideally, if performed by two or more people, the bold lines will be read by everyone, and the other lines will be read in turn by individuals. The script is a linear play of Timeline 1. As you perform and hear it, please keep in mind that time is not a line.

Silence has a presence.

Silence is a dominant force within the history of AIDS.

Silence is not absence, or lack of sound.

Silence is what could happen but doesn't.

In AIDS before AIDS there is an emptiness. There was nothing known about AIDS to be silent about. The First Silence begins in 1981.

A *New York Times* headline about a rare cancer seen in forty-one homosexuals.

A report about babies born with similar symptoms.

A poster hung by a nurse in San Francisco about "Gay Cancer."

These utterances happen around the same time.

But not together.

Silence is a lack of connection.

Silence is known when it breaks.

The First Silence breaks when Ronald Reagan himself breaks.

Reagan's refusal to say AIDS in public was not the only silence.

We could not have gone from the First Silence to AIDS Crisis Culture without suffering, action, and words. Silence is never alone.

Silence is always paired . . .

. . . with frustration, loss, life.

. . . with solitude, introspection, curiosity.

Within silence power can be and is born.

The Denver Principles were written in 1983. The People with AIDS Coalition was founded in 1985. The First Silence.

Treatment Action Campaign in South Africa begins in 1998. The Global Coalition on Women and AIDS was founded in 2004. The Second Silence.

Within silence, people find others looking for connection.

So much is missed in silence, including the not doing, the not connecting.

Silence breaks open.

Silence recedes slowly.

I emerged from silence.

I made a break from silence.

We could not have broken from AIDS Crisis Culture to the Second Silence without medication, hope, exhaustion.

I think the Second Silence was clarifying.

I thought that silence was going to be the permanent state of AIDS.

I was lost in silence.

The violence of silence is that it stalls the flow of ideas.

I'm not sure when the silence ended, or if it ended. In some communities silence is still rolling, swirling, and then clouding over.

We could not have gone from Silence to Revisitation without time.

From Silence to Revisitation is a call and response.

From Silence to Revisitation we witnessed pain.

From Silence to Revisitation we witnessed the past in the present.

From Silence to Revisitation we witnessed trauma together.

We could not have moved from Revisitation to Normalization without confronting trauma. The Revisitation worked. It took AIDS into time.

Normalization is based on abundance. Silence is quieted by Normalization.

After so much silence, it can be comforting to see AIDS normalized.

Normalization can feel crude and confusing and banal.

HIV sits among other viruses.

AIDS gains its place in history.

In Normalization AIDS [crisis] is condensed, hidden, real.

AIDS crisis and silence never disappear.

We will always have silences. We will always have viruses. We will always have conversations.

PART TWO
SILENCE

7 SILENCE + OBJECT

TED: A lot of time passed between the creation and distribution of "Grandma's Legacy" in the early 1990s and when you found your dub of the work in your collection of VHS tapes a few years ago as part of our research.

ALEX: Something like twenty-five years. But this feels huge not only in terms of the many years and stages of my life, but more so, if we think about the life of HIV in culture. So much happened in those years between AIDS Crisis Culture and when we began to engage again with the Bebashi video during the Revisitation. We both lived through a long and hard period of quiet. The Second Silence. The quiet seemed so ominous and horrible after the noise and activity of AIDS Crisis Culture.

TED: As someone living it, I just assumed that this would be the state of AIDS forever. It felt simple, wrong, and also immovable. Over the years, we have generated a functioning definition of the Second Silence, but that has been hard.

ALEX: Overwhelming.

TED: But wait, before we get into the definition, and progress from there, can I just unburden myself with something I want to have recorded in our conversation, but that we don't need to get into?

ALEX: Sure.

TED: Thank you. Over the years, I have been thinking about, tracking, and growing a list of all that I think has been impacted by the Second Silence, and the ways in which it is still ongoing, even if the silence has been broken. Silence impacts:

- experiences of diagnosis pre- and post-1996.
- collective HIV history, memory, and meaning-making, specifically the tactics of surviving, thriving, and dying with dignity that is cultivated by voices that have been minoritized within the AIDS response.
- the role of AIDS service organizations and the shrinking place of community.
- the role of AIDS service organizations and how AIDS went from a public and community concern to a private, medicalized concern.
- the disappearance of discourse on the impact that AIDS and related treatment has had and has on the experiences and bodies of people living with HIV.
- the reception and circulation of art created in the twentieth century about AIDS.
- the reception and circulation of art about AIDS created in the twenty-first century.
- how we make sense of the disparities in who gets AIDS-related care, be it in the form of treatment, representation, or culture.
- the relationship between gay men and HIV, and between gay men themselves because of HIV.
- how AIDS is being and not being written into US and world history.
- the location of the onus of the epidemic: from being shared within larger communities, to being put solely on people living with HIV.
- stigma, discrimination, and criminalization.
- the stories we tell and don't tell about HIV.
- the amount of time it took for undetectable to be communicated in a meaningful way.

ALEX: That's quite a list!

TED: I needed to express it as a way of letting it go. It is and was too much for me to hold alone.

102

ALEX: Happy to help. But I think we can all gain from this. By detailing silence's multiplicity and immense impact across a range of registers, your list serves as an invitation for me, and also our readers, to enter the conversation. Everyone can pick a bullet point and do their own deep dive: imagining the shape, impact, and feeling of one aspect of silence or another, just as we are about to do here. For every one of us each aspect of silence will be known and felt differently.

TED: I am ready for that process, for us and them. I can't muster the strength to do it all alone.

ALEX: Your list makes clear that silence has a presence, or actually presences; a gravitational pull or pulls that is bigger than the present. It subsumes the present.

TED: Agreed. If our object in Part One was the Bebashi tape, then Silence is our object in Part Two.

ALEX: How weird is that! Ted, silence isn't really an object. You can't hold it, or really even share it. It's more like a state, or an event. An affective condition that you suffer through or fall into or get locked within. It is a mode of being not an object. Sometimes we choose it, but more often it finds us. And if we do choose it—which perhaps is true for me and many others at the beginning of the Second Silence—I certainly didn't choose for it to last as long as it did!

TED: I hear you. Let me say this differently, then. Before we begin to give words to some of the many competing moods, states, hopes, and pains of silence— our focus for this part in the book is illuminating silence through conversation.

ALEX: Yes, Ted, and this is hard. I know we each had our own silence. But for people of my generation, the heart of our silence is an awful darkness. A terror or a grief and an anger. Another kind of death—even while living—that is amplified or itself mirrors the actual bodily deaths of so many people during the Time of AIDS it follows. Silence does not exist alone. Silence always has another part, and its most brutal sister is death. Silence = Death. Death will and must always haunt AIDS work, at least until we get to some fantastical and also sort of creepy moment in the future when no one is honoring their dead (or worried about their own mortality in the face of HIV). What does death mean within the ongoing production and reception of AIDS cultural production?

TED: This is a question I think we should leave open, with an understanding that all of our responses, if not directly related to death, are part of the answer. Death, as you say, is always in the conversation when we talk about HIV. At the same time, I want us to push forward, because as I have come to learn, silence is not just the bedside friend of evil or annihilation. Silence can be judgment-free. It can relate to good as much as it protects bad.

ALEX: While I know you are right, I also feel like you are being evasive, or maybe just shut down. But then again, when engaging with people of your generation, who haven't lost a close friend or lover, it's not like what I want from the Revisitation is to make you share or even suffer my pain or loss. And given that HAART ended up working really well for many people, Silence itself also changed and has grown to hold (new) life: for those whose prognosis changed, and for others who never experienced their HIV as a death sentence.

TED: HAART did usher in more life and also activity into the world of AIDS. And this is also a little confusing. Because the irony is, after 1996, with less death and better health, there were more people living with HIV than ever before. And yet by our own calculations, that is when the silence around AIDS settled in again, anew.

And actually, I want to push back. I have been part of the AIDS response for twenty years; of course I have experienced multiple deaths, of people I knew well and loved, and people who have been important and influential to me, and of course, strangers who I am connected to. Now, and throughout the Second Silence, there are—and have been—deaths. But to your point, the overall thrust of AIDS culture changed to center around "living with" (and maybe that is why, in part, there is this idea that people my age and younger have not experienced AIDS-related death). So what you have named as shutting down, is maybe just another way of being with.

ALEX: But because of the Silence—and associated treatment and medical advances—the very act of living and being "with," as you say, took up less space in public, just as did death. Memorial services and other forms of commiserating for someone who died used to take up a lot of space.

TED: I can imagine. And for me, what I have noticed is that the visual space that people living with HIV once had in culture—specifically gay and lesbian culture in the late 1990s and early aughts—has diminished. Side effects of early medication disappeared or changed. Encountering people in our daily life with sunken cheeks and deep smile lines (facial lipoatrophy), or big bellies (lipohypertrophy)—both side effects of AIDS meds—started to happen less as medications improved.

ALEX: And part of the hard and painful work within Silence, at least for those of us who remember that earlier time, but more so who remember those people, is a sense of duty, a burden to tell and retell, share and reshare what and also who was.

TED: Which is what ended up happening later, after the Silence, in the Revisitation.

ALEX: Right. The Second Silence is what happened as we were all holding the burdens of memory, duty, suffering, on our own, in our own way, and in isolation.

TED: Second Silence is the lack of circulation, even as AIDS was still ongoing. People received new diagnoses, some died, and others were saved. Within the Silence there were also huge strides forward. For instance, there was a significant reduction in vertical transmission (what was once known as mother-to-child transmission); spending on AIDS increased globally; progress was made in relation to treatment; PEPFAR was created during the Second Silence, as was research into PrEP. In the city we live in, and in many others around the world, government and health services for people living with HIV became better, not worse. And movies were also produced, artworks created, babies born, books written; organizations were founded; scientific advances were made.

ALEX: But even as there was production and possibility, the feelings of loss, confusion, and contradiction remained. And for those who were now living healthy lives with HIV, AIDS continued in other ways—for instance, as a memory or threat—and these too became less visible or discussed: interpersonally, institutionally, and throughout the media ecology. In regards to media, I also struggled at that time with a feeling that the baton of representation was not being handed off. Not only did I not know who to past it to, but worse still, I was not sure anyone even wanted it.

TED: This is one of the tricks of silence. We can't hear or sense what other people are doing or even wanting. So in fact, I was that person wanting to grab and carry on the baton. But because of a variety of factors, including lack of proximity because of silence, it took time for me to find you and let you know this; it took time and energy to connect.

As I will detail more in the next chapter, during the Second Silence I was volunteering and then working at HIV Edmonton, an AIDS Service Organization in my city. It had to move many times in the city over its long history, always due to financial reasons as well as stigma, because nearby businesses and organizations were uncomfortable with the people we served, primarily people dealing with HIV and homelessness, and mental health, as well as a significant client base of Aboriginals against whom there is significant bias. But what binds all the HIV Edmonton locations in my mind is the huge amount of stuff each office had.

ALEX: What do you mean by stuff? Computers? Needle exchange supplies? Condoms?

TED: Yes. But what stays with me, and what made an impact on me then, were the boxes of old AIDS Walk t-shirts; folded up memorial AIDS quilt panels; containers of old photographs from white-tie fundraisers, ribbon cutting ceremonies, and outreach events populated by people I recognized from the office and other people I knew to be dead; official proclamations signed by previous city mayors; used candles from memorials; books of signatures from memorials; flat files of posters from over the years and around the world; boxes of old videotapes, some of which were in professional big black plastic cases and others in flimsy paper boxes written on in pen; and paintings, so many paintings of red ribbons, young people crying, and wild animals. The paintings were often the most upsetting to me, even more than the photos because they were the most obviously connected to people's experiences of emotional pain. All this stuff was packed together, taking up so much space, sometimes entire rooms. The once vibrant world of AIDS that I had been called to seemed to be both hidden away and stuck there. But I also couldn't look away. I was interested and invested in the objects' former public life. I started to wonder, what purpose does AIDS culture serve when people stop paying attention and things get boxed away?

ALEX: It's true, so much of the inspiring and useful things we worked so hard to make during the period of AIDS Crisis Culture somehow went missing within the Second Silence. The amazing, productive Bebashi video is just one example of countless such tapes that went and are still hiding in plain sight: the people who made them are still around, the boxes they are stored in are still available. AIDS Crisis Culture went dormant in the Silence. And this includes all the posters, drawings, books, essays, photographs, and poems that we had made to save each other's lives. My friends and I have some of this stuff: art and ephemera in filing cabinets and storage units. Under our beds. In small boxes of mementos. In our closets. We moved the diaries and letters, clothes, and art of friends lost to AIDS across the country because we

106

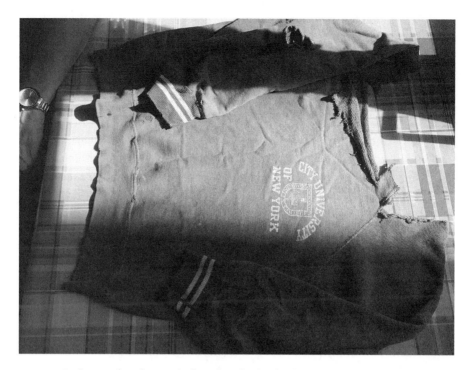

7.1 Jim's sweatshirt, bequeathed to Alex after his death in 1993. Given to Ted in a healing ritual needed as a result of writing this chapter in Ditmas Park, Brooklyn, 2020.

would never throw them out. And the Revisitation has prompted many of us to engage again with those collections. My VHS Archives project tries to address what to do with my boxes of AIDS tapes, for instance.[1] I engage in this project in a working group of others (including you) who are invested in tape, AIDS, archives, and activism.

TED: The ongoing life of AIDS activism ephemera is the subject of our final chapter in this part, "Silence + Transformation." *Metanoia: Transformation through AIDS Art and Archives* literally emerged from the boxes of two women from your generation who were engaged in AIDS Crisis Culture in California: Judy Greenspan and Judy Sisneros. Each had recently donated some of her collection of AIDS activist artifacts to a queer archive.

ALEX: It has been so moving to hear them both talk about the burden of those boxes, and also the relief of handing them over to the ONE Archives in LA (Judy Sisneros) and the LGBT Community Center National History Archive in NY (Judy Greenspan). Many of us are finally beginning to make sense of our personal collections. *Video Remains*, which we will discuss later, is my early attempt to make sense of one of my own boxes that holds a dead person, although in this case the box was the black plastic casing of a VHS tape holding fleeting images of my best friend in the months before he died of AIDS. This painful process of navigating the very culture we made in the face of mass death, only a decade or so later, feels like it has no historical analogy.

TED: Comparisons could be made, but I am not sure to what effect. AIDS is not like war, or even like other health outbreaks. There is something specific about its mass death, cultural production, and stigma that makes dealing with what HIV leaves behind unique.

ALEX: That isn't just about me and my generation, Ted. You've made quite a bit of stuff, too. A good deal of it during the Second Silence! What have you done with all your boxes?

TED: I don't have a lot of boxes. A lot of my stuff lives digitally. Also, I left my city in my thirties and chose to leave behind a lot of things. And I haven't accumulated much since. I am not good at safekeeping.

ALEX: You are saying the things themselves don't matter?

TED: No! I am saying that for better or worse, tending to what we are calling "my boxes" is not something I have done well. And in that, your point is well taken. Of course, I have a history, and that history has material consequences and residue. What does it mean to be doing AIDS work for so long, and not have boxes? What aren't I accumulating or saving? And maybe, to play arm-chair therapist for myself, what does my lack of boxes have to do with the rooms of AIDS past ephemera that I encountered as a young person doing this work?

ALEX: I must admit that I feel a kind of displacement or projection happening here. Like, I'm the person who has to have the boxes, and the grief, and the duty, and the burden, and then do the work to make sense of it later and pass it on, which leaves you free and clear to, well, I'm not sure to do what. Maybe you don't have to have history and pain if I carry it for you?

TED: I think we could write a whole other chapter, if not book, on your last line, this idea that younger generations are more free from suffering due to the people that came before. And I think that idea is something very alive within AIDS cultural production, including activism. I am not sure how alive it is between us. To abstract us for a second, I think there is a tendency in

108

any cross-generational conversation rooted in AIDS for there to be a privileging of stories from the 1980s and early 1990s. But I want to say that this is as much about deference, and cultural habits and norms, as it is about any hang-ups I might have about my own pain. Then, to get back to us, my intention is not for you to be the holder of pain. Yet I see the impact of my words on you. I think that while I am processing my past in my own ways, I am not paying attention to what I am placing upon you about your past.

ALEX: Mine is big and yours is small? Mine is hard and yours is easier? Mine is old and yours is fresh? That sort of thing? I am stuck and you are free?

TED: No, I'm not saying that. I don't even mean to suggest any sort of one-sidedness. I think maybe there is something in what I am saying, and in what you are receiving that is highlighting our own kind of stuckness.

Pause

Speaking for myself, perhaps silence—and talking about all this with you—provides a way of seeing those rooms of stored AIDS Crisis Culture as a literal embodiment of the silence around AIDS, one that I was confronting and struggling with. On the one hand, proximity was comforting, but on the other hand it was frustrating because the life of the objects seemed so, I dunno, far away. It wasn't even like a museum exhibition that I was invited to consider but never experience . . .

ALEX: I think I know where you are going with this: those objects were a connection to the past you never got to live. And I get that. As someone who has been asked to play the "elder," I have negotiated a lot of spaces with people who want to know what it was like back then. But believe me, it won't be too long before people want to do projects on *your* "old" projects. That strange sense of temporality often haunts our interactions. Sure, *AIDS TV* is "old," but much of it is still utterly pertinent, and useful. We're basically writing segments of it again. We're relooking at many of the same tapes and coming up with similar (and new) findings.

TED: AIDS is not primarily about the past for me. It was (and is) about the present.

ALEX: Again, I'm going to have to ask you to reconsider what you're saying here. You've created a shell game where I must represent the past, I must suffer loss, I must account for my past, and you are somehow "not interested in the past."

TED: Thank you for naming that. And again, we find ourselves trapped in this script of intergenerational AIDS dialogue that is not rooted in what is true about you, or me, or our relationship, or process. I will offer some context.

Pause

Let me say that it is not that I am not interested in the past. Rather, I am ambivalent about the past as a motivating factor for my work. I understand that I need AIDS history to do AIDS work, and I am grateful for it. What I would say, and I hope we talk about this more later, is that I don't feel displaced in time. I am not a gay man who wishes he could have had sex in the 1970s. I am not an AIDS activist who wishes he could have been with you and others at ACT UP meetings in 1987. I am not a feminist who yearns for some sort of more ideal and radical past. (All three of these refrains being something we hear often in our community.) Rather, part of what coming of age in the Second Silence did for me was to make me grateful for the times I was in, interested in the times from before, and excited about building with others times to come. And maybe in this way we are alike, and that is what makes the shell game that tries to contain you in the past so unfair. You, I think, are also a person of your time, at all times.

ALEX: Thank you. I feel seen and also like I understand you better. I am glad you aren't nostalgic for my past. I'm not either! Today is good. And we have a lot that we need to do now. Because, of course, beyond a kind of joie de vivre, we also share AIDS, and there's a lot of work to be done to make living with HIV a joyful or transformative experience.

TED: And we share that as young people—in very different circumstances and times—AIDS became an organizing principle in our lives, for the reason you express above. So again, to speak for myself, I had strong feelings when being faced with physical signs of an AIDS reality no longer being dealt with. The AIDS Crisis Culture stuff that was left behind was not even being treated like trash, because at least we deal with garbage by taking it out. Instead, these physical connections from the recent life of an epidemic were not even being touched, catalogued, used.

ALEX: Okay, I respect that you didn't know what to make of all the goods that were left behind, but I can tell you that at the end of the day, objects are just things. Focusing on them misses the depth and space of loss. Jim's 80s puffy cowboy leather jacket, which I wear on occasions to this day, reminds me of him (and me) at that time. It puts me in physical proximity to something he touched. But it's not a replacement or even a substitute for him: a person. That's why, also at the end of the day, I'm a process person. Our conversations and interactions sustain me; as mine with Jim once did. And that's why, for me, our book is about times, states, and methods, using objects to help to get us there, to help us to live. Certainly those objects are redolent with feeling, ideas, meaning, and processes, and they give us so much. But mostly, they open out our present to ourselves, and to others.

TED: I think there is a difference between the stuff I am talking about and what you and your friends have held on to. Maybe I have been messy and conflated the two in this discussion. A major difference between Jim's jacket, and the rooms I keep coming back to in this chapter, is the personal. Even if you never wore Jim's jacket, even if you hung it in a closet and did not look at it for twenty years, his jacket and your relationship to it are different from what was happening at ASOs during the Second Silence. At the very least, we could say the difference is around registers of grief: that of a person mourning a person, people, and a time; and that of an organization overwhelmed by grief, work, bureaucracy, and not managing their shit.

ALEX: Ted, can you ground this in something? Would a person, object, or feeling help you?

TED: Sure. I have some experience bridging these different registers of grief because of my time at Visual AIDS, an organization whose mission includes helping to promote, salvage, and share the art of people living with HIV. In 2011, while I was still just interning there, Chloe Dzubilo died. She was a long-term survivor with HIV. She was also an East Village legend who did amazing activism, was an important performer and rock star, and was famous as a muse. A few months or a year after she died, bins and bags and boxes of her artwork, and some personal artifacts, came to Visual AIDS. Eventually this was moved to the Fales Collection at the NYU Library. Before that, the space that her materials took up encompassed a lot of VA's small one-room Chelsea office. But the spiritual space it took up was even larger. And it wasn't just because she died. It was also because there is a real weight to her brilliance and therefore her things. Those boxes and bags were filled with some of the most funny, meaningful, and insightful works on paper I have had the pleasure of engaging with about HIV. We are so lucky that power of her work adorns and enfolds our work as this book's cover. To say nothing of the collage with the pink feather, the binder full of glamour shots of her taken by Alice O'Malley, and other important photographers.

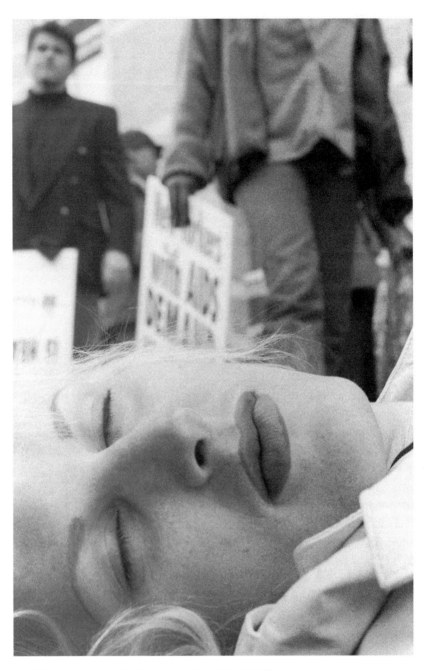

7.2 Chloe, ACT UP Die-In, New York City, Alice O'Malley, ca. 1994.

Sure, it was at times inconvenient to host a condom-stuffing event, or interview volunteers, or welcome school groups to the space maneuvering around the objects of a legend, gone too soon. But never once did any of us at the office want Chloe's stuff to just disappear. Nelson Santos, the assistant director at the time, eventually reorganized the office so we could coexist with the stuff a little bit better. But once it left, the space felt empty.

I say all that about Chloe because her stuff in the VA office is much closer to Jim's jacket in your apartment, or even on your body. While you held on to Jim's stuff in the quiet storm of the Second Silence, Chloe's memory as well as her work has become important within the Revisitation. There is an emotional resonance that comes from how their objects were saved and tended to. This is very different from those rooms back in Edmonton. The difference is around what gets abandoned, what gets too overwhelming to deal with, what gets brushed aside. That can happen to a person and on an individual level. But that was not what was of interest to me as a young person. I was taken in by the collective and shared abandonment of AIDS.

ALEX: Thanks for this detail. Listening to you, and learning with you, I can now say that the similarities between Jim and Chloe's stuff are also around what these saved objects prompted us to do. And remember, the shame and pain of the Second Silence is about not managing those things—and they are not tchotchkes, they are talismans.

Revisitation happens when (at last) we confront our objects, but really our people and our feelings. Part of what clicked in my burgeoning relationship with you at the onset of the Revisitation was your interest (and mine) in turning things into events, encounters, experiences. Core to your AIDS work was a drive to activate encounters, where before and still (in the Silence) people had been isolated, maybe locked in all alone with their things, and worse still, other's things. This meant building new spaces that were rich in possibilities for feeling, and sharing, and passing on, and by definition, where the emotions in the room would be as disparate, competing, and hard to express as have been ours here. I am not sure if you ever did a Chloe event per se, but in hearing you talk about her stuff, I recognize an impulse to not only save, and care, but also animate and share: to do with and from the things. This is why I am so very moved by her images on the cover of our book!

TED: There have been many Chloe events. Even a quick look at the Visual AIDS website will steer someone in the right direction to learn more about her and her life. As for what you were saying, something amazing to see is when the physical weight of things—a life, art objects, archives—takes on a new kind of weight as cultural production, as conversation, as shared memory, as book cover. I love seeing that those boxes of stuff are what allowed for Chloe's artwork to now be curated in gallery and museum exhibitions. I so loved being in a room full of people watching the sweet punk rock footage that Kelly McGowan took of Chloe being used with love by Viva Ruiz in her Visual AIDS commission video *Chloe Dzubilo: There is a Transolution* (2019). I think that urge to take the isolated stories and also things of AIDS, then to build around them some space so that they can be shared, is something we have both been called to do: to help break silence.

ALEX: I must admit that I did not exactly feel *called*. I feel more like I called, and called, and called, by myself—using video—and no one answered. Until they did. And that calling provided a space for more calls. Throughout the long silence, each call was different as well as isolated. While you were wondering where the AIDS present was, my experience of the Second Silence was more than disorienting: it was painful, bleak, and mortifying. It was not just objects that got lost, friends that died. I got lost. I suffered survivor's guilt. I blamed myself for not staying active and true to the cause.

TED: Is this what you and your cohort were feeling during the Second Silence?

ALEX: I can't speak for anyone but myself, but it seems to me that there were lots of Silences, just as there were so many of us: some of us were breathing a sigh of relief thinking that if AIDS itself was not over, the worst of the crisis was; others went from working at ASOs that went from well-funded to under- or un-funded; others still were traumatized, isolated, or confused. And then for some, the Silence marked an end.

TED: So the Silence, while being many things, was also a reprieve?

ALEX: Maybe at first. For a while, it felt like a necessary break from too much noise, action, engagement, or illness. It was a reasonable response to fatigue and PTSD for those who had experienced so many deaths, including surviving their own. Things can't be at crisis pitch forever, by definition. To nurture your own health across an ongoing event of AIDS demanded a scaling back.

TED: Meanwhile, the beat of the world continued. People were getting the internet in their homes; another Bush was in office; attention on the World Trade Organization brought new life into an emerging generation of activists with a different orientation to crisis; and people were fighting like hell to head off what was to become decades of perpetual war in the run up to the Iraq invasion.

114

ALEX: Yes, but also, there are feelings connected to those moments.

TED: Millennium fever was followed by the dangerous mess of 9/11. And since then, it has felt like a litany of impending crises have dropped on us, like climate change, war, or immigration. While AIDS was never a single-issue concern, it was a huge tent that dominated social and political landscapes.

ALEX: For so long in the Second Silence AIDS felt private, something to manage at home, on your own. After 1996, when we gain meds to treat the virus, a movement basically packs up and is replaced by business. Silence=private. As is true of many movements during this period of neoliberalism, the collective spirit of the AIDS response—as activism, volunteerism, institution-building, care, or cultural production—ceases to be primary, visible, or productive of more. And even though it is true that for many AIDS is and was suffered as a personal psychosexual concern, during the previous period of AIDS Crisis Culture we had worked hard to characterize and operationalize such personal experiences as communal and political concerns. That is why the silence— that is to say the lack of connection—was such a cruel thing to live through once it began. After AIDS Crisis Culture I felt my own experience of activism, and that of the Left more broadly, to be more fractured. I was still showing up for the world, but within the morass of issues, AIDS was showing up less, and then less again.

TED: Right, and I was witnessing HIV/AIDS as an unseen part of the world. So while one part of my life was informed by stockpiles of AIDS cultural production from the past, another part was clocking the evacuation of special AIDS episodes on primetime TV or new work in queer film festivals.

ALEX: I witnessed the evaporation of large demonstrations and actions in which some people found community; support groups and activist meetings for the uninitiated were harder to find; galas and cultural events to raise awareness and money, and also to network, occurred less and less for and about people living with HIV; there would be one screening of AIDS work at yearly queer film festivals, where there had recently been so many.

TED: Along these lines, perhaps we could think of the Second Silence as a time that came and then also continued as a more subtle lingering, unfolding, staying, and dying out.

ALEX: I don't know; mostly I felt tired and stuck and sad. For my generation, a lot of people we love died. *They* died out. But we had planned to save them.

That was what had inspired us to work: to make art, noise, community, and infrastructure. Activism inspired by people dying is particularly extreme and intense. The person that you love is egregiously ill and in pain for months, years. And for most people in the AIDS community it wasn't just one person, it was their community. It's a truism of activism that things don't happen as quickly as you want them to. Over the long haul, people ran out of stamina and then feel bereft.

Pause

But for people in my generation, you can only say that so many times until you feel like you're stating something that's self-evident, or boring, something that everyone already knows. But every time you say it, it's real again to you: "I was an activist because people I know were dying around me." Then, a cycle of quieting begins internally: "Why am I even talking about this now? Are we going to talk about this again?! I can't keep rehearsing my pain in public or even as an act of politics." That's another reason why people silence themselves. We stopped talking about AIDS because everything had already been said, and one generation's pain cannot sustain a movement, or really much of anything.

TED: This is yet again another moment of our divergent experiences of this same period. I can't match the emotional load that you are carrying.

ALEX: And I don't want you to.

TED: I know that you don't want me to. But it is not that easy. The Second Silence was confusing because silence produces a sort of self-fulfilling prophecy by which individuals think they are supposed to be quiet. If no one else is talking about AIDS, the thinking goes, then maybe I shouldn't either. And there is also the external idea that no one wants to hear it, otherwise, there'd be more talking. I have often failed to ask about HIV with someone because they have not brought it up first.

ALEX: This dynamic, although maybe respectful, is no way to break through silence. It also is not very empathetic. This is why we have to talk about how we feel, what we need, how we can be together in difference. This is why we need careful, caring, conversation about AIDS. Objects help.

TED: Right. This is something filmmaker Hayat Hyatt explores in his 2015 short experimental film, *Villanelle*. As abstracted, collaged, and moving images move across the screen, we meet a small group of Black gay, queer, and femme men talking about community and connections in the context of their lives. Among the voices is an older Black male interviewee. He shares with us the phenomenon of hanging out in cross-generational gay spaces and not feeling able or welcome to talk about HIV/AIDS with younger gay Black men, as if it is too depressing or too long ago to be of interest to young people. It is heartbreaking to witness; he is holding on to his pain in isolation. This moment of his reckoning is a powerful and heartbreaking illustration of the Second Silence. We see the gulf between what we get from hearing his testimony and the fact that this man felt he had to create a silence, at the cost of his own happiness, to protect others in his community.

ALEX: The sad truth being that younger people, like Hyatt, and like you, were living in silence too, and desperately wanting conversation. Hence the video. While some of us needed and wanted to be coaxed out of our silences, some of us did the coaxing. I think it is critical to implicate you in this, even if you have a different relationship to grief and trauma. One's age or generation does not link in a one-to-one way with when you are ready or able to break silence, connect, make demands or requests, or create friendship.

TED: One thing that is not clear to me is to what extent you and your friends tried or did not try to coax each other out of the silence.

ALEX: Ted, why don't you talk about you and your friends? For me, the silence was for some time about self and community care. Until it wasn't. That's when I made *Video Remains*. I initiated conversation within my community and across generations.

TED: Alex, I am not asking you questions in hopes of not having to answer them.

ALEX: But by now you must understand the dynamic it produces.

TED: Yes, of course. By not talking about my pain, my community's losses, and the silences I am part of as they are connected to AIDS, we are producing a conversation that suggests none of that is alive in my life, in the life of my friends, in my generation. And that, again, is not my intention. And it is not true. The thing I hate most is AIDS culture that treats the crisis like a thing of the past. But here I am, as you are suggesting, reproducing that. But I am wiser about how and why that happens. Can I dive in a bit more?

ALEX: Please. I am learning. I know this is hard. Maybe we are revealing or working through some gendered, as well as age-based, roles we've been playing together and not attending to until now: about who has feelings, and who reveals. I want to be clear, we both get something from that dynamic!

TED: Maybe, and the gender thing is real. I also want to say, we are upending some expectations as well. In some ways time has moved fast in the last few years. I have been in rooms that are almost opposite to the world Hyatt brought us into. AIDS of the past is the dominant discourse, and no one else can speak besides those who were there earlier, unless invited to connect to what is already being said. And that creates a different kind of silence. We have friends, of various ages, who became positive within the Second Silence and even more recently. They face a specific and terrible stigma from the AIDS community. This is distinct from the shared stigma, criminalization, and discrimination that all people with HIV face. There is a lack of empathy, of grace, and a kind of cruel confusion about how someone could seroconvert in the twenty-first century.

So I agree with what you said earlier, about how one generation's trauma cannot sustain a movement. But there is a way in which the many versions of silence have created the conditions in which we are often trapped about how to see each other and our movements.

ALEX: Pushing for shared vulnerability—across time and difference—takes intention, and trust, and some discomfort. As we have discussed, we are often currently in rooms talking about AIDS where we will not know the HIV status of the people around the table. And we understand why that is. Stigma is real. An ongoing impact of the Second Silence is that there is still uncertainty— even within the AIDS community—about where it is safe, appropriate, or necessary to disclose one's HIV status. No one wants to be the only one, no one wants to be tokenized or deferred to, and no one wants to be the first to ask. But it is worth saying that knowing and sharing our positive, negative, and unknown status was something that I experienced in the past as a way to ensure that AIDS was rooted in all times, and within the conversation. This was core to AIDS Crisis Culture.

TED: HIV is a material reality that is in some people's bodies, and that has real impacts on people's lives; at the same time, experiences of AIDS, including its burdens, are something that can be shared.

ALEX: If the conditions allow. There has been something so important for me about sharing the burden of AIDS with you (and then others as we publish). I remember life during the Silence. I'd come across a listing for some AIDS-related event and no matter what it was, I would make the effort to attend.

Sort of like what I used to do when a film was directed by a woman, or lesbian, or person of color. The difference of course being that in the thick of the Silence, the audience would usually be less than a handful of people—yes, happy to see each other, but also despondent and maybe retriggered by all the indifference. Would we ever be in a warm room again filled with people united by HIV?

TED: When you go through an archive of someone involved in the AIDS response, you inevitably find clippings of newspapers and magazine articles about the end of AIDS, or wondering where the movement has gone. This is how you realize that the preoccupation of my own early AIDS experiences, and our work together, is shared by many of us in the AIDS Response. For example, Gabriele Griffin wrote a book, published in 2000, *Visibility Blue/s: Representations of HIV and AIDS*,[2] in which she wrestles with the public visibility of the crisis. Writing from inside the Second Silence, she one-ups us. She eschews the word "silence" for "re-invisibilization," making the case, just as we do now, twenty years later, that the history of AIDS is marked by periods of seeing and unseeing the crisis.

ALEX: My friend and our colleague, the recently departed Douglas Crimp, wrote about this in 1989. In "Mourning and Militancy" he does not use the word "silence" per se, but he does say, "the turn away from AIDS can be seen as one response to the epidemic from the moment it was recognized in 1981."[3]

TED: This is a profound way to talk about not saying or seeing. As we have been fighting the virus, we have also always been fighting the silence around the virus.

ALEX: Douglas was so important to the movement, and to me personally. So smart, and refined, with and of us. I miss him now because he is silent, just recently rendered so through death. Yes, I can read his writing and we can talk about his work, but he can't keep working with us, or being with us, teaching us. So let's think about what his words mean and more: every turning away from AIDS leads to a turning to. Every silence initiates a sound. Every stillness helps to inspire an action. Maybe not for any one person, but for our movements.

+ OBJECT

7 SILENCE + OBJECT

1 **SILENCE + YOU**
Set a timer for one minute. Use that time to sit in silence. Afterward,
record your thoughts on the experience.

2 **SILENCE + OTHERS**
Try the above exercise with another. Share your thoughts.

3 **SILENCE + THE WORLD**
Two readings about silence and AIDS:
- Kathy Boudin, ed. *Breaking the Walls of Silence: AIDS and Women in a
  New York State Maximum-Security Prison*. Woodstock, NY: Overlook,
  1998.
- Avram Finkelstein. *After Silence: A History of AIDS through Its Images*.
  Oakland: University of California Press, 2017.

8 SILENCE + ART

TED: We both came to our personal understanding that there was a Second Silence because we each felt it on our own, alone, but also in our separate ways.

ALEX: With this in mind, Ted, before we focus on your artmaking and activism during the Second Silence in this chapter, turning to what I did during this time in the next chapter, are you okay with doing an exercise together? Will you share with me more personal associations that come up for you when you think of the Second Silence?

TED: Yes. Let me take a breath. Okay: industrial carpet in an office. Isolation. Excitement. Awareness about the future and knowing that there's more than is readily available.

ALEX: Thank you. And trust that we will come back to this in our conversation. Now say more about that office, which I assume is related to the storage closets you spoke about in the previous chapter.

TED: Yes, exactly. It is HIV Edmonton, where I first was able to find HIV community and where I ended up working in the early 2000s.

ALEX: Less timeline, more impressions.

TED: Okay. It is midday. None of the lights are on because the ceiling lights are too bright. The windows are big enough that the natural light of midday is nice, but it keeps everything in shadows. I can see the office where Trudy, the volunteer archivist, sat, right in front of the windows in front of the city. She came in on Tuesday and would plunk herself amid almost twenty years of banker boxes. These boxes have a different charge than the objects I have previously mentioned. They are being touched, tended to, cared for.

ALEX: Wow, intense! And good. Say more about that mix of isolation and excitement. And those boxes. Are the feelings and the boxes both in the room at the same time?

TED: Same time. I'm a person who's interested in something that most people are not—AIDS—and that's really isolating. But I know that I'm doing something of value and I'm excited about connecting.

ALEX: Good. Thank you.

TED: Okay. Now it is your turn. Give me some impressions.

ALEX: Breakfast. Silverlake. Late morning. The light is very California bright. I've had the right amount of coffee, so I'm feeling lively. I am meeting Pato Hebert for the first time socially. Today, these many years later, he's our friend who is an amazing artist and educator: an AIDS worker of the best sort. With him, at brunch so many years ago, there is an electricity of connection.

TED: Explain that. Can you give me more feelings?

ALEX: I associate that time, that breakfast specifically, with positive and also negative emotions. And pleasure. The pleasure of connection. So much of the Silence is about the lack of connection, about a fear of foreclosure around what I am allowed to discuss. Meeting someone who I think is brilliant and also interested in the things I am in ways that are exciting to me because he will take me to places I haven't been for a long time. But that's also shameful.

TED: Why shame?

ALEX: If you are asking for my impressions of the Second Silence, then much of it is that I don't deserve to be talking about AIDS cultural activism with a peer, that I am not sure I have peers anymore, or that I am no longer a peer (or an AIDS worker). So shame for what I don't know, don't do, haven't done, can no longer do.

TED: Okay. Last feelings or impressions?

ALEX: A sense of curiosity which begins to emerge as familiar and sustaining, but not mine to claim. Yet.

TED: Thank you for that, Alex. That was meaningful; it left me with a sense that we have a lot to talk about.

ALEX: Yes, because silence guts the present of its presence so we have to speak to know silence.

TED: True! During the Second Silence it was important for me to find a way to make AIDS in the present visible, tangible, or operational for myself and others. I realize through our process of conversation that my urge to connect led me to make as much content as I could about AIDS. Here's one of my favorite creations, a postcard I made in 2012 when Lana Del Rey was at the height of her cultural ubiquity.

ALEX: Huh? Help me out here. Generation and pop culture gap . . . I don't even know who she is!

TED: Lana Del Rey was the go-to diva-in-training for a generation of gay boys, queers, and other navel-gazers. She had a 2012 hit song, "Video Games," that was dreamy, sad, and danceable. She came on the scene as a twenty-first-century sex kitten fit for Elvis, and ripe with her own obvious insecurities and imposter syndrome. At the time, if you were young-ish and hoping you were at least beautiful in an outsider way, then Lana was your girl. I was drawn to this mix of a nostalgic figure in the present who took up space on the national stage but was signaling to the weirdos, queers, and others, whose name and presence I wanted to use in a work.

ALEX: But she isn't HIV+ is she? Does she even sing about AIDS?

TED: I don't know the answer to either of those questions, but at the time of making the card I am not sure that I cared. I was frustrated and tired of AIDS being associated with the past. Like I mentioned, unlike many of my esteemed peers, I am less connected to AIDS of the past. For as long as I can remember I have wanted the crisis to be understood in time, not of a time or out of time. Part of what the Second Silence felt like for me was being in a world built on AIDS but with no real acknowledgment. My image was one way for me to circulate AIDS in the culture, grounding the experience of the virus in the present.

ALEX: What do you mean, a lack of acknowledgment?

TED: There was no culture being made at the time about HIV that was circulating in any meaningful way, beyond the stuff created by ASOs and the

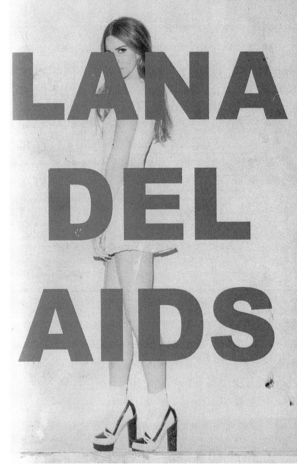

IN THE SHADOW OF THE EPIDEMIC:
Being HIV-Negative in the Age of AIDS

Walt Odets

For gay men who are HIV-negative in a community devastated by
AIDS, survival may be a matter of grief, guilt, anxiety, and isola-
                                                          hate look
                                                          e lives of
                                                          perience as
                                                          issues,
                                                          denial,
                                                          fected gay

                                                          t are
                                                          sexualtiy
                                                          al ques-
                                                          st of
                                                          irecting
                                                          ntial to
                                                          ful first-
                                                          the need
                                                          epidemic's

                                                          ctice in
                                                          f the Gay
                                                          well-

8.1 Lana Del AIDS, postcard series (2010–ongoing), Theodore Kerr.

government. But that didn't count, it all felt like public health messaging, not the culture. So in response I made visual noise. I collaged her "now"-ness with a now-ness I felt for AIDS. And I knew her brand could absorb the association. Maybe it might even be made better for it among some of my fellow fags. While I wanted everyone to pay attention to AIDS, I really wanted those who I called "my people" to pay attention. I wanted us to be publicly wrestling with our cultural inheritance of AIDS in the way I now see younger generations doing. Lana, I felt, was the perfect image to help with that.

ALEX: We will always be so different in this regard, Ted. The way I knew how to make AIDS visible was to show it in its utter, glorious, particular vivid difference from mainstream culture or life. The funky alternative worlds in which AIDS is lived.

TED: We're not so different. And I don't do anything that other mediamakers in the AIDS response haven't done before or are still doing. For example, My Barbarian is an art collective made up of Malik Gaines, Jade Gordon, and Alexandro Segade who, in their own words, "use performance to play with social difficulties, theatricalize historic problems, and imagine ways of being together."[1] Their work is often about AIDS, like their video *Counterpublicity* (2014), a performance made in relation to José Esteban Muñoz's essay about Pedro Zamora, AIDS activist and star of the *Real World: San Francisco*. They, along with the visual arts duo PRVTDNCR & BODEGA VENDETTA, and critic and curator Emily Colucci (who loves Lana Del Rey with an unmatched ferocity to mine), are some of my peers who see pop culture as a helpful vehicle for talking about AIDS.

ALEX: Granted, national or international media do dictate, to a large part, the public's understanding of AIDS. But Ted, let's not forget the intimate media scale of "Grandma's Legacy." Its earnestness went lost too.

TED: That's one reason I love that tape and was so glad we found it! I am so earnest on a daily basis that I annoy people. But with that in mind, I have no skills to make earnest art. Like, what would I do, make a postcard that says, "Think about AIDS. Now"?

ALEX: Yes.

But let's not get stuck in a generational trap about cynicism and earnestness, or mainstream or alternative culture. We both live now, where those binaries have collapsed.

TED: The level of earnestness and depth that I want and crave from AIDS work is something that *was* done. Today, it is received in other ways, as is only to be expected. You and your friends did that work, in that way, back in the day. I think much of your analysis and politics has aged well. And because of that work, I didn't and don't have to go there or do that. I wanted to point to it, and drag it forward, but I feel and felt no need to duplicate those truths already so well stated. The urgency I felt and feel is in the lack of contemporary context when it comes to AIDS.

ALEX: So let's pause to be flat-footed for a second. You only knew about the work that we made because you were looking.

TED: Yes. I was using the internet, but not only. I was going to the library. I was talking to people. I had a boyfriend back in Edmonton who was a painter, and in school he learned about General Idea. He was excited to share their work with me. And like all nerds, anything that struck my fancy became a tunnel to more.

ALEX: The work from the past you were consuming was not stuff that was readily circulating?

TED: For the most part, no. While I was in Edmonton, I helped run a queer culture festival and as part of that work I was part of the national queer film scene, where many programmers locally, and across the country, were helpful in pointing me to films I could watch and program. It was also through those connections that I learned about DIVA TV, and met Tom Kalin. In fact, if I think hard about it, there is a good chance I saw some of your work long before I even knew what I was looking at or for.

ALEX: So you weren't ignoring alternative work. You were curious but not in deep-research mode. And like we said earlier, one of the main functions and strengths of popular culture is that it makes alternative culture obscure, difficult to get to, irrelevant because pop culture is itself so big. And to return to some of our thoughts from the last chapter, you are saying again that the past was a consideration but not central to your work in the present of the Second Silence.

TED: AIDS was important to me but my work was not only about the virus. During the Second Silence, I was deeply excited about being an adult, an independent gay adult. So the work was as much about my politics and a reflection of my research as it was the world I wanted to make and the person I wanted to be in that world. So that is why Lana makes it to the postcard,

126

and not someone more obvious like Britney or even Madonna. I was crafting a queer contemporary response to AIDS within a world that seemed utterly void of it, and maybe disinterested. I found this exciting because as a young person I believed in my own power of persuasion; I thought I could convince people to get on the right side of history with me.

ALEX: Say more.

TED: I get the sense that you learned about HIV/AIDS in real time as the crisis was first unfolding, and you—people you know and your friends—also helped shape what would become the culture of HIV in response. So as a young adult, HIV and the response, and your own making of the response, shaped you. I imagine that for you, AIDS was defining, if at first discrete. It was separate from life before.

ALEX: So true. All of that. When people of my generation (and older) talk about this break, we usually do so around sex: like, "Remember when you could have sex and not worry about getting a life-threatening virus?" But what you're asking me to think about is more fundamental than sex. I was changed by AIDS not because I acquired HIV, nor solely because I worried about that possibility, but because AIDS made a break happen, which kept happening for quite awhile, in how I lived, loved, thought, and made art. And then there were more breaks that kept on coming at me. Our rough periodization doesn't simply mark the changing quantities and topics of AIDS cultural engagement but also structures of feeling, living, and human interaction that changed noticeably in cultural production and then also in me and others. That's why "AIDS is over" has never made any sense to me on a personal or a political level: I'm defined by it, and I helped define it, and that changes, as do I, which feels powerful at times and brutally disabling at others. For AIDS to be over, I'd have to be over.

TED: And while it is true that I, too, have experienced, engaged with, and been changed by the different Times of AIDS cultural production, my encounters are different from yours. There was no discrete time before AIDS for me. Rather, I grew up immersed in AIDS Crisis Culture. I was a young and susceptible consumer, a gay boy within the period in which you played an active part as a producer. I was taught about AIDS in school, and I worked hard to get my hands on any magazine devoted to AIDS that I could find. But by the time I was a young adult in Edmonton, all of that was gone. While I did not have the historical vision or language, on some level I knew the Second Silence had begun because my generation was coming into adulthood in a

127

vacuum where AIDS once was and was now basically absent, and in this way also everywhere. This was particularly true for me because AIDS was in my mind and my psyche, in a very loud and formative way, and yet there was no place to see it reflected back at me in public. That is, in part, why I brought myself to the ASO in Edmonton. Does that make sense?

ALEX: Yes. I remember looking into the world during the Second Silence and not seeing my own interests or history reflected back. I like how you describe this. But I'm curious: Why was AIDS so central to your formation, even as it was invisible? Is the answer as simple as the fact that you were a young gay man coming into your sexuality and adulthood?

TED: Yes, but that's hardly simple! As a young gay person, it was ingrained in me that HIV was "my issue," that the virus and crisis were my cultural inheritance. While for many of my peers this meant that HIV was an inevitable medical and social condition they would contract, for me, AIDS was like a road map to adulthood.

ALEX: Wow, say more about that.

TED: Okay, so even though I grew up in Canada where gay marriage was legal for most of my adult life, my idea of gay was very not heteronormative. Being gay was about creativity and experimentation, a kind of freedom across time and space that was not connected to single relationships, be they sexual, emotional, or otherwise. And I knew to build that life would take time, and because of that I wanted to be thirty years old more than anything. I wanted to have an apartment and a vast array of friends who were living out all of our cool life stories and pursuits. And this vision of a scintillating gay life came not from my family, but rather from the people slightly older than me who I met while working fashion retail. And also, of course, from the culture. It was from these sources that I learned how to be a thirty-year-old, independent, queer person. And the lives of the people who shaped me were directly and indirectly shaped and dominated by HIV/AIDS.

ALEX: Growing up, your definition of being a gay man was a person impacted by and responding to AIDS. So you were looking for people like me!

TED: Exactly! And in time I have come to see that my version of who and what this person could be was different from what most gay men my age aspired to. Many of them also understood adulthood through the lens of AIDS, but in a way that made them afraid of it: either because they might be a victim of a premature death due to an HIV diagnosis, or a victim in the sense that by coming after the plague years they had missed out on some sex utopia that I have never really bought into.

ALEX: Right. That version that says the tragedy of AIDS is sex with worry or likely death.

TED: And that wasn't my story. By my own admission, I was a sexless teenager, and I knew enough about myself and HIV to know that I was less at risk of contracting HIV than others. And coming into adulthood, I was certain there was a community of AIDS-aware and gay adults just waiting for me and only slightly out of reach. I was so eager to join them.

ALEX: For sex, community, identity?

TED: All of it! That is the hubris of the young, I guess, because when I finally made my move and started to volunteer at a local ASO, the situation was very different from what I had imagined. The gaggle of hip adults I had seen stationed around the registration desk at local AIDS walks in the 1990s, looking so cool in their free shirts and clipboards, flirting and laughing, were nowhere to be seen. The room full of witty handsome gay men and sophisticated and urbane women that I had seen in films like *Parting Glances* (Bill Sherwood, 1986), and even *It's My Party* (Randal Kleiser, 1996) were nowhere to be found. That version of the AIDS response was over by the time I arrived. In its place was a group of people who have always been part of social change, and were always part of AIDS cultural production. However, these activists are seldom pictured as being part of HIV/AIDS: women of color, lesbians, Two-Spirits, people who do drugs, people who live in and fight against poverty, radical left white people of various sexual orientations and genders, and of course, well-meaning liberals.

ALEX: The very people we are or have become as well as those that our shared work centers! But at the time, you were disappointed?

TED: Yes and no. At first I just didn't understand. I was excited and overwhelmed by everything I was doing and everyone I was meeting. I didn't have time to consider what I was missing. And in the back of my mind I was assuming the people I hoped to meet were actually still around, and I would happen upon them the next time I was in the office. Or, when I was there long enough, I would bump into them. That moment never came.

But I wasn't disappointed. Quite the opposite: I am grateful for who was there. Previously to volunteering, I had a very narrow idea of who was impacted by HIV: it was gay men, women in Africa, and other people (this undefined but open category of people who I could not exactly name because they were rarely if ever shown). But turns out, it was actually this group of others, wonderful people all, who were running the organization! Through them I was able to grow into an intersectional awareness of HIV that was informed by a First Nations, Two-Spirit, immigrant, feminist, feminist of color praxis of HIV that understood the virus to be one of many issues facing people living with it.

ALEX: Well, interestingly, that's my story too, just for different reasons, and grounded in another time and place! I came to AIDS through these same people—wickedly smart, already highly able activists who had refined their tactics via feminism, anti-racist, anti-war activism; those sixties people in the AIDS movement I so admired—and their sets of approaches toward an intersectional analysis and activism. As a young, college-educated feminist, this was how I was taught to see the world, and I (like so many feminists) brought this to a brand new political, social, and bodily phenomenon, AIDS: a systemic analysis of oppression that linked violent systems as well as empowering responses.

TED: The number one issue for people who accessed services at HIV Edmonton was around anti–First Nation bias, as well as homelessness and poverty, and their connections to stigma around drug use and mental health. HIV was a real issue, but it was also another way to access services when other doors were closed. I did not meet a gay person living with HIV until years into my work, and that was one of our board members. From there, it was not until I went to a retreat across the country, in 2006 maybe, that I met people my own age with HIV.

ALEX: And here's one of the places of deep disconnection between us: the person I knew best who was my own age and had HIV died of it at the age of twenty-nine. Jim and I came into AIDS together. He was a gay man. I was not. We were both changed by AIDS. Jim died. And I was transformed by his death.

TED: And I think that difference is one of many conversations that people need to have cross-generationally, across class, across experiences within the Second Silence, and beyond. Within an intersectional understanding of HIV, there is still an urgent need to include gay men. And in some ways HIV Edmonton saw me as a way to do just that, to not lose the gay men we loved, the gay men still living with HIV, the gay men who might never get or would be treated for HIV. They sent me to national meetings about prevention efforts for gay men. But also within me, a white, cis-gendered gay man who was part intersectional feminist warrior, part lez-bro, there was still a need to connect with gay men who were not unyoked from HIV. I also needed to connect to men who were at least as tethered to the virus as I was, and this is where my first Second Silence art project came in.

ALEX: Tell me all about it as another way to get into your silence.

TED: In 2007 or so, my friend Marshall Watson—artist, project manager, writer, and musician—was bemoaning with me that the representation of gay men in the media was limited to depictions of us as childish sexual objects, and we decided we could make our own representations better. So he was the first subject of collaborative portraits that I started doing of queer dudes in their underwear in my apartment. The underwear could be used in any way they wanted. Some just posed, enjoying their beauty; others got a bit more creative with props or characters; and others really just used it as a moment to think about how they wanted to be represented.

ALEX: Honestly, I am drawn to their eyes and less their garments. And why underwear if you were trying to get away from stereotypical representations of gay men?

TED: Ha! Right! So maybe I was sexless as a teenager, but by the time I was in my twenties I was less sexless. Also, in terms of creativity, underwear started off as a wink and a nod at the high rate at which gay men are pictured solely in their underwear.

ALEX: And these guys have on underwear but also so much more, and by that I don't just mean garments. They have on their connection to you and their own personal brands of humanness.

TED: Thank you for that. I have spent years kinda embarrassed by this project because of how basically horny it is. But when I look through your eyes, I remember, and I am able to own and claim that so much of this project was about seeing and being seen by gay and queer men. So yes, we were young, and near naked, and flirting. And in that, we were also connecting, sharing, being vulnerable, and curious. AIDS did this for us.

ALEX: AIDS "did that" for us, too. Our world was flirty, sexy, and charged. Living in a plague did not stop us from caring about what we wore, how we looked, our attraction to other people, how we made art about and with each other. Maybe it even sharpened it. But Ted, how exactly did AIDS do that for you and Marshall, given that it had gone missing?

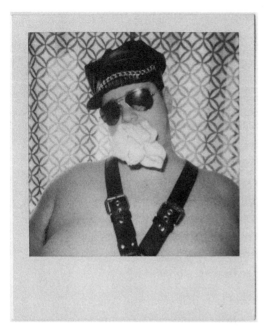
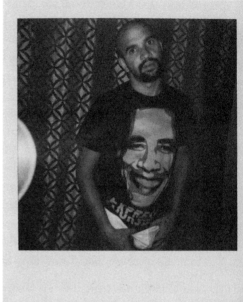
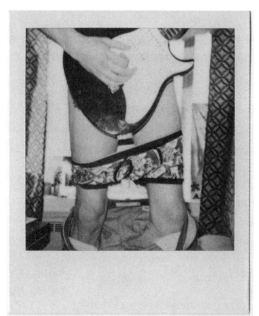
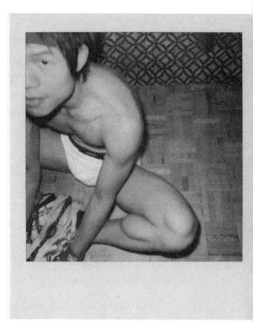

8.2–8.5 Polaroids from Kerr's "One on One" Project (2009).

TED: Part of being curious and annoyed about how gay men were being represented at the time was contemplating how this came to be. This eventually led to us thinking about the impact AIDS had on a gay aesthetic. I think I summed it up best during a talk I gave around this time in Edmonton about how the mid-twentieth-century image of gay men was frail, old, and creepy. In the 1970s, with *Three's Company* and *Soap*, gay men were starting to be seen, but primarily as comic relief and harmless. Then, with HIV/AIDS we were seen as frail again, and also young, tragic, to be pitied and helped. In response to HIV, gay men and those who wanted to market to them pictured us as young still, but also strong, and innocent: that is to say, illness-free and uncorrupted. It was this last phase that Marshall and I were dealing with. We were part of a generation of young gay men who, like anybody, wanted to be seen as desirable ourselves, within a lineage, but also on our own terms. We didn't need or want to be seen as super-fit or overly sexualized or even overly safe or dangerous. These were the main categories of gay male representation available to us. We wanted to break out.

ALEX: And because of the timing of it, you must have also been dealing with the internet, online images, and digital influences.

TED: Yes, what Marshall and I were doing was part of something bigger that was being impacted and shared on the internet. The growth of personal computers and smartphones meant we had unlimited images at our fingertips, including the rise of influencers, and porn. So there were forces of the past and present weighing down, and exciting opportunities for communication and self-representation opening up. It was a time of strife and tenderness, mediated by the twentieth century and the World Wide Web. The result, I thought, was the development of the "Soft Queer gaze," a visual language created and used by queer gay men that blended domesticity and the erotic. It is on full view in films like *Weekend*. You can see it through the objectification of the intimate and the stranger in Paul Mpagi Sepuya's work, and with a real desire to confront subjectivity as explored by both *Butt Magazine* and *Original Plumbing*. We wanted to be sexy, seen, and available, but also soft, kind, and building toward something; marking, or at least debating, ideas of permanence, because this was when we could start to have online profiles that we could use to court friendship, sex, and other opportunities. There was a lot of hand-wringing around how cruising would soon be a lost art due to Grindr, Jack'd, and Scruff. Less were we negotiating the implication of clones, and more were we considering how to market ourselves in an online space in an attempt for connection. Around this time open relationships

133

within gay communities started to get discussed more, as did throuples, and the creation of bespoke and social justice–minded pornographers and porn stars. And on some level, all of this is on view within the Polaroids I took with my friends. There we were negotiating visibility, body, and desire.

ALEX: And history.

TED: Totally. Not only the weight of history in terms of understanding our bodies as political projects and signposts of progress around the rise of medical advancements and emerging prevention technologies, but also tactics. So maybe cruising on the street was being replaced with apps, but the strategies we used on apps were shaped by the images that were created earlier. I used Polaroids because I had learned that in previous eras, including in the early days of AIDS, queer people would use Polaroids to create their own representation free from the prying and often censoring eye of film developers. Trans women would capture their looks, gay biker gangs would trade pics, artists and pornographers would make and sell work. By taking Polaroids, I was both engaging in a process of transparency (allowing the men I was photographing to see the work as it was being made), and I was also recalling older ways of being gay and visible in the world.

ALEX: Looking at your work also reminds us that while same-sex desires have always been fraught, the anxiety of sex for gay men in the twenty-first century cannot be uncoupled from HIV/AIDS, even in periods of silence around the epidemic. I can't imagine that it is possible that your sexual love, domesticity, desire, and artmaking wasn't always aware of HIV.

TED: Right, and that came out in the process. In almost every case, a guy would come over, I would make him tea, we would talk at my counter for a while about life in general. The conversation would work its way to the photo and from there we would begin to talk about our bodies, desires, fears, and hopes as young queer men. What always came up was HIV/AIDS, and specifically fears and questions that the guys had about HIV and the role it was playing in their ever-evolving sex lives. In part this was because this was what was on their minds, but also it was because I was associated with HIV/ AIDS. I had used my status as one of the only gay people at the organization to make a case that it was a welcoming and wonderful place for gay men. And this was something supported by the organization. At some point I went from volunteer coordinator to the "Artist-in-Red." The "Red" here refers to the ubiquitous ribbon. This was a totally made-up position that allowed me to do art-based programming to bring in an audience of my peers. And it

134

worked. I made film screenings, and workshops, and community discussions for gay men (and others).

ALEX: Ted, I just want to name something here. As much as you are talking about your work, you are also sharing a lot of ideas that you seem to have been carrying with you since back in the day. This is not a criticism, just something I wanted to name.

TED: That is a good point. And maybe this is a good example of what is made possible by taking time to be in dialogue with someone, getting to know their past motivations and desires, getting comfortable and better known. This can be as much about the important subjects at hand as it is the submerged knowledge that emerges.

ALEX: What interests me in what is coming to the surface now in your story is that even when no gay community easily or obviously presented itself to you, the connections between them, and you, and AIDS *was* there, and you found or you made it through art and interaction. You were addressing a particular silence within AIDS and the Second Silence: that of gay (white) men. I say this because maybe another key to understanding the reach, power, and particularities of the Second Silence is to take account of this critical absence that you experienced. I am not sure this gay exodus is universal, but it was something real for you and your friends.

TED: Around the turn of the century, there was a reconsideration of gay men's place within the AIDS Response. I witnessed this on the local level as the lack of gay people at HIV Edmonton, but it can also be seen in other ways. The introduction of life-saving medication made more explicit the class divides that had always been present within the epidemic. These exist along racial, ableist, and behavioral lines as well. For many gay men living with HIV, the introduction of medication addressed and ended the crisis. But for immigrants, drug users, poor people, and others, the fact of the meds was one step toward responding to AIDS but not nearly enough. There were issues of access and adherence, what we in Canada easily refer to as the "social determinants of health." The World Health Organization refers to these as "the conditions in which people are born, grow, live, work and age," and the long list they use is informative and reminds us that this is the part that is not easy: income level, educational opportunities, occupation, employment status and workplace safety, gender inequity, racial segregation, food insecurity and inaccessibility of nutritious food choices, access to housing and utility services, early childhood experiences and development, social support and

135

community inclusivity, crime rates and exposure to violent behavior, availability of transportation, neighborhood conditions and physical environment, access to safe drinking water, clean air and toxin-free environments, recreational and leisure opportunities.[2]

ALEX: When you put it this way, it seems hard to forget that AIDS has stayed present as a condition of poverty and racism as much as it is connected to sexuality, sex, and sexual identity.

TED: Right, you can see this play out when some gay men living with HIV and other gays no longer felt comfortable accessing services at the very AIDS service organizations they had used, or invented, during AIDS Crisis Culture. In the Second Silence, there might suddenly be issues of hygiene in the lobby of these places, active overdoses happening in the bathroom, and institutional priorities moving away from gay men and toward other identities. I know from my work in Edmonton that gay men felt they had built these organizations which were now being overrun by communities they did not see themselves being a part of. In Vancouver you saw the founding of HIM, and in Seattle you saw the founding of Gay City Health as a result of these feelings: separate gay male health spaces that receive AIDS funding and are specific in their outreach. While much is made about mainstream attempts to de-gay AIDS, less is made about how that is not totally unrelated to the ways in which some communities of gay men tried to de-AIDS themselves when AIDS became too associated with other communities, and when they got meds. Nothing I am saying here is groundbreaking to anyone working in the field. If you have been doing frontline AIDS work even for a minute in the last twenty years, the divide between the white gays with money and access and everyone else is as clear as day.

ALEX: It was true in the past as well. At that time did you already have these critiques, including your thinking about the absence, silence, and presence of white gay men? And if not, what were you doing to figure it out? And maybe hardest: How do you think about your own place within this, given that you were visible as a gay white man working in AIDS at the time, and in all Times of AIDS?

TED: I was heavily influenced by a project called Against Equality started by Ryan Conrad and Yasmin Nair that took the shape of blogs, books, stickers, and social media presence.[3] They were my generation's answer to Queer Nation. They critique HRC (Human Rights Campaign), and other projects of homonormativity. And it was within that work that I could see the weight

136

of the gay male connection to AIDS. While I could see activism including an intersectional approach in my local community, the popular imagery coming out of the United States at the time was around marriage, army recruitment, and representation. Even though Canada has its own issues, our activism was still often heavily influenced by what was happening in the States. So something like the AE postcard series was helpful. It reduced the cruel glare of what we may call Gay Inc. and created, at least for me and other people I knew in Canada, a kind of cross-cultural queer solidarity.

It was around this time that I started the postcard project that Lana Del AIDS would eventually be a part of. The idea was to create an art project that mirrored the epidemic itself—that is to say, materially-based and circulating. The first set of images I made was rooted in wanting gay men in the city to see HIV Edmonton as a resource for them, specifically around agency, negotiation, and safer sex practices. I got some money to print cards created in collaboration with different artists. On the front was a photo taken by my one-time boyfriend Zachary Ayotte of the two of us, plus a story I wrote about a sexual experience I had in Spain, a failure of communication. Then on the back is an illustration of how to put a condom on with your mouth.

ALEX: Ted, we started with a trust exercise of sorts. Will you engage with one here as a conclusion to our learning from your stories within Silence? What did making these cards, given how personal are their images and stories, do for you personally, as a young man in the Silence?

TED: AIDS gave me life, purpose, friends, a way to see the world.

ALEX: Me too. Including you.

TED: That's the good part. But it has also given me frustration, loss, and much pause around who I am, how I am, and my place in the world. AIDS is my life's work, which makes sense because one could argue that the work done in response to AIDS has made my life possible.

8 SILENCE + ART

1 **SILENCE + YOU**

What are artworks—visual, music, movies, video games, literature—that have helped you see AIDS or HIV more clearly? Find images.

2 **SILENCE + OTHERS**

Using the images from above, share them (in a meme or postcard like Ted did, or another format that you feel comfortable with).

3 **SILENCE + THE WORLD**

Here are three examples of arts communities breaking the silence of AIDS:

- The Keiskamma Trust: a German/South Africa community arts partnership that, among its multiple programs, uses art to address issues of poverty and HIV: http://www.keiskamma.org/the-keiskamma-guernica/.
- PosterVirus: a Canadian/US collaborative project of public art and AIDS: https://postervirus.tumblr.com/.
- Visual AIDS: an organization that utilizes art to fight AIDS by provoking dialogue, supporting HIV+ artists, and preserving a legacy: http://visualaids.org/.

9 SILENCE + VIDEO

ALEX: Thanks for sharing with me how the Second Silence, for you, was about figuring out how to get involved and identity formation. For me, it was about reentering AIDS in the face of loss. I think it is no accident that in our previous exercise you conjured up the presence of Trudy, the archivist, while I conjured up Pato Hebert, the AIDS worker par excellence. Both, while being real people, are also stand-ins for our own human need and hope during the Second Silence. Now, I see new points of connection.

TED: Like what?

ALEX: How we each engaged with AIDS during silence. Coming back into a way of living and contributing and interacting that I thought I would never do again. The sustaining life practice that I had left behind.

TED: What do you mean?

ALEX: I mean that while I was busy and doing many things during the Second Silence, none of them were AIDS-related. Meanwhile, here was Pato—in all his present busy commitments and tasks and energy around the epidemic—revealing to me the world that I had been missing, longing for, and that I thought was gone. The world of AIDS in the present.

TED: Right. On top of his work as an artist and a professor, Pato was working for AIDS Project Los Angeles (APLA) at the time.

ALEX: Yes, and he still works for the Global Forum on MSM and HIV, to help organizations strengthen civil society and push governments to better meet the health needs and human rights of LGBT people.[1] I was captivated by just what Pato embodied so authentically in the middle of my own silence, and the larger one we are trying to draw out here. This is what left me gob-smacked at brunch. I was busy with my new life in LA, but the past was hanging over me if now also hidden (by me), a looming reminder of something I was not doing, not seeing, no longer knowing. I wanted an AIDS worker in my life. I wanted to be an AIDS worker again, but no longer knew how or where I could be this.

TED: But I don't understand why you weren't just doing it.

ALEX: I come from a generation who in the face of AIDS built local, activist, rag-tag responses, remedies, ways of helping, and reacting: AIDS Crisis Culture. As time and the epidemic marched on, most of those things became either professionalized or silent. By the time I moved to LA in 1995, I felt really alienated from the AIDS response because it had become something else, and specifically, I guess I would have to say, corrupted.

   I get it. We need systems in place to allow for treatment. But with that comes a related reduction of nuance. Cut off from an intimate view of the crisis after leaving New York City for LA, my understanding of HIV during the Second Silence was that the only work that was being done, and maybe that needed to be done, was being executed by "AIDS Inc." And yet at the same time, I knew this could not be entirely and fully true. I knew that there must be more work to be done, that was being done, because I knew that I needed it. The AIDS crisis, while not the virus, was still in me.

TED: I can imagine for you that the Second Silence was less about connection, as it was for me, and more about reconnection. How did you do that?

ALEX: The way we always do even if it doesn't always click or hold: looking for and also making art and culture helped me loop back and forward. In 2005, I ended up making my first AIDS video since the early 90s. It was about the Second Silence, although I didn't know those words yet. It was about coming into words and connection again, so also breaking through my own silence with others.

TED: You are talking about *Video Remains*?

ALEX: Yes. Part of what I wanted to talk about with Pato was what would eventually become *Video Remains*, a project that had been percolating inside of me for a while. Sometimes active, itchy, tantalizing, and other times heavy, quiet, present. I was going to finally do something with a piece of videotape that I had saved, not looked at, and carried forward from my past with AIDS.

TED: *Video Remains* builds upon what can be known after the unspeakable—another kind of silence—by watching and listening to you talking with people left after a tragedy. One could say it is an attempt to begin to unpack the individual and collective silence and trauma of mass death, loss, neglect, and maybe even one's own actions taken.

ALEX: I ended up making space to visit that trauma first for myself, and then also for my contemporaries, who I interviewed in the video, and then for audience members as much in need of this as we were, using what I think of as an ethical, communal, known interaction within and about the Second Silence. But first I had to figure out how to do all that and then the words had to be coaxed out.

TED: So let's engage with your video, and its processes—much as you did with your peers—as a way to model archival care, and get into the heart of the silence you were trying to leave.

ALEX: I will go to the past, with you, and *Video Remains*. But I have already written and spoken a lot about *Video Remains*. And I already went, rather painfully I must admit, to my past to make that video. Now we are visiting my visit of my past: twice over! Your reading of my writing about the tape is how you first found me on the internet! It inspired our first conversation.[2] If we are going there again together, I hope to break new territory with you: personally, conceptually, interpersonally.

TED: I'm excited to try. This seems like a safe place to experiment.

ALEX: We'll see . . .

TED: I'm really interested in what motivated your work, how it felt, the inner workings and processes of silence and also breaking through it. I can ease us in. Your video begins with sweet footage of you and James Robert (Jim) Lamb walking up the stairs of a typical New York City building to your apartment.

ALEX: Six flights! Our six-floor walk-up on Attorney Street. It takes a good long time to get there . . . and I tape the whole climb. We lived there together for many years. It's only just now being gentrified!

141

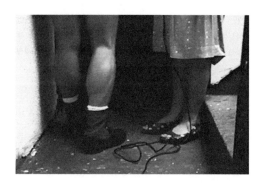

9.1 Jim and Alex's feet outside the front door of their Attorney Street apartment. Still from *Video Remains* (1990).

TED: You are sexy and in love with each other the way that only young people who are buoyed by each other's existence can be. This unspooling piece of video acts as an introduction, a glimpse into the domestic friendship that you must have had.

ALEX: When I watch it again, I love that there are two bumper stickers on our front door: one about AIDS, the other about reproductive rights. And I always wait for when the door opens and I get to have a glimpse of our apartment—its brown and tan colors and still so familiar furnishings—as well as our young tight legs, standing there together at the threshold. I loved those red polka-dotted platforms and of course Jim was in his so-80s combat boots. But I also run sound of me talking on the phone with my friend and fellow AIDS video activist, Ellen Spiro, under this unedited take. I explain to her (and the viewer): "You understand what I'm doing here, Ellen? I'm making a video about the near past and the present specifically in relation to AIDS." I tell her I'm going to revisit some haunted footage I've been holding onto for years: of Jim, in that time, and about his death, and video.

TED: From there, you cut to that footage that you took of Jim on a trip in the early 1990s when you visited him in Miami. It plays for almost an hour in close to real time, intercut with footage you shot after the fact, in the early aughts.

ALEX: In 1991, I had left Jim and New York and was living in Philadelphia. I missed him (and New York) so much! I flew to Miami to shoot him for a video that we were ostensibly making together. But at this point in his life he was pretty deranged—either as a direct result of effects of HIV or perhaps AZT to his brain, or as a reasonable psychological response to dying of a disease in his late twenties when there was no cure and a great deal of pain.

142

TED: The raw footage from the original tape is primarily Jim on the beach talking . . .

ALEX: And the sky and ocean so blue behind him. Talk about VHS! The hues are depleted and enraged in equal measure. I was using the same camcorder I bought to make the WAVE tapes.

TED: The tape ends with the two of you in a hotel room.

ALEX: You can catch the only image of me in the tape with Jim in the mirror there (I also show up in another mirror, too, caught in the reflection with a different man, Michael, my hair stylist. I cut that interaction into the original footage of Jim when making *Video Remains*). And then, from the original tape, you see that I took a few short shots of the mid-century hotels from the outside, in the dark, as I was leaving town. And then the original tape fades to snow. This image also ends up serving as a metaphor in the piece I would make from it.

TED: You tell me that Jim is rambling and not himself. Some viewers might pick up on this, others will just see a slightly loopy handsome young white man, facing death (or not), and trying to carry life with him.

ALEX: Maybe some will identify a certain sort of 80s theater queen (now mostly lost to us, too, both from death and changing norms of gay male behavior), which would be true. Jim was a successful downtown actor in the last years of his life, working for Everett Quinton's reenergized Ridiculous Theatrical Company after Charles Ludlam's death from AIDS. For the Ridiculous, Jim was almost always cast as the stupid beefcake, although he was both erudite and educated (we met in college at Amherst). In the footage, he still is beautiful although perhaps not as well-spoken as he imagined. He was a really handsome man. Famous in the East Village for his looks (and his unexpected quirky demeanor, given his outward presentation)! But at times during the tape he gets sweaty or his ear or throat hurts and he suddenly doesn't look so good, and he tires over the tape's real-time hour. In his life off the tape, up until the last few months, he kept his visual appearance mostly together. He got so much pleasure from being admired and wanted. Of course, I remember how terrible he looked at the end. My unrecorded visions of his decrepitude haunt me as much as do any I saved on video or photo.

TED: Before we keep tending to the tape, let me ask an obvious question. What made you start the project?

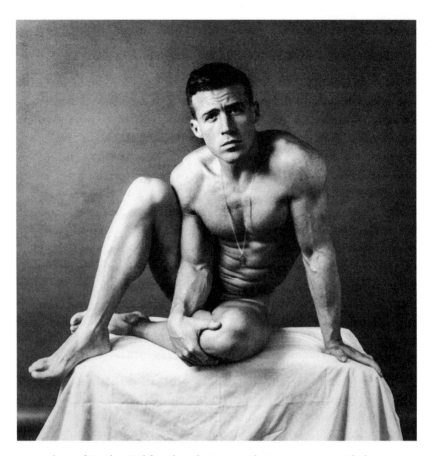

9.2 A photo of Jim that Ted found on the internet during our retreat with the Quakers, fall 2019. © Victor Carnuccion.

ALEX: I came to *Video Remains* because I was feeling, well, silent. But also, sad ... it was a way back to Jim. Jim, my best friend, my "boyfriend." Jim with whom I had sought to understand adulthood. Jim who I would explore the world with. And Jim, who died, and whose life and death I think about all the time, and whose memory I feel a responsibility toward. This was part of the shame that I was holding on to when I met Pato. If 2000s Edmonton for you is about figuring out how to be an adult, a gay male adult, then 2000s LA for me is about being a full-on domestic woman: raising kids, dealing with romantic relationships, and balancing home, writing, and a full-time and demanding life of teaching, making, and being social. But suddenly this was all happening, for the first time in my adult life, with AIDS *not* at the center. But

144

always with Jim there too, buried but live (and dead), and thus feeling that I was letting him down.

TED: By not remembering him, as you have suggested?

ALEX: Well, yes, but no. More so, for not doing anything about AIDS. It is not that I thought AIDS was ever over, but I had positioned myself very far from it. And as we are trying to make clear, discussions about AIDS that were certainly happening in LA were not reaching me, even though I was only a circle or two removed. And maybe this is because I wasn't looking. This to me is my silence deep at work. Other noise and my quiet being so close to each other, and yet so unable to touch.

TED: But somehow, the noise came back for you.

ALEX: As we said earlier: maybe static first? A buzz. An itch. A confusion. A bad tape, sorta like a bad trip or an actual bad trip (to Miami; that was sad and also held things I wasn't ready to deal with. Who would?). In any case, I was finally ready to deal with that tape of our weird and painful trip to the beach and Jim's performance on it. This was also a way of saying that I am ready to deal with AIDS, and ready for AIDS to deal with me. Again.

TED: Yeah, I like that: ready for AIDS to deal with me. I spent a lot of time in Edmonton waiting for AIDS to deal with me, and while I was waiting, I kept on dealing with it myself, taking up any AIDS-related invitation that came to me from coworkers, and bringing my friends along with me or making a space where people who wanted to talk about HIV could do so around me. This is what you were doing in *Video Remains*. Interspersed within the video vessel, your actual trip footage, you end up cutting in new vignettes: such as your conversations with kids from MPowerment, the youth group you were invited to attend by Pato, at APLA.

ALEX: Maybe that's why I use the images of snow (as a transition device between scenes) and embrace the initial tape's VHS glitch. As smooth as some of my transitions are (I actually blend Jim and the kids from APLA when I transition between them to both visually and politically connect them), I also want there to be some jarring interrelations.

TED: You move from Jim on the beach, talking, to scenes where we see queer youth of color, mostly but not exclusively Latino or Black and male, younger than you were when you met Jim. They talk about AIDS, and sex, and relationships, and fear and desire.

145

+ VIDEO

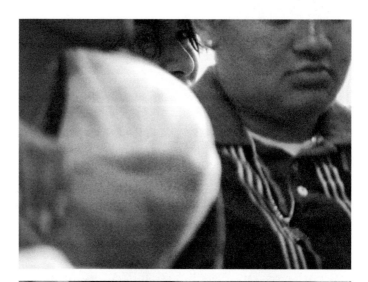

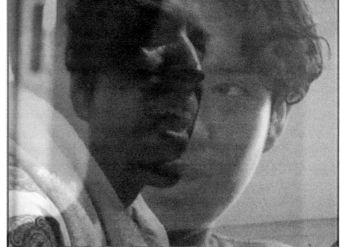

9.3–9.5 Collage
of screen grabs
of Mpowerment
participants from
2008 footage by
Miquel Angel
Garcia and
Alexandra Juhasz.

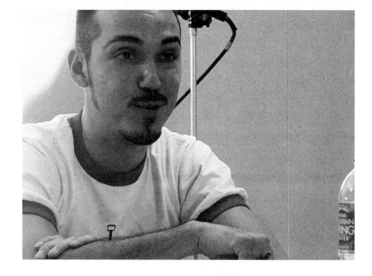

ALEX: Right, this is where Pato comes back into the story. At that brunch in Los Angeles, I told him I had an AIDS project that I wanted to work on, and asked him if he would help. I explain that I don't know how to break back in because I've been gone for so long. I'm not sure I should. I explain parts of what will go on to become *Video Remains*, talking to him about the footage I have of Jim that's been sitting on my shelf for ten years that I'm haunted by, that I have a responsibility to, that I don't know what to do with, that I feel so bad about. It's all negative to me. We were in Florida, Jim was not well, and I didn't always feel connected to him even as or because of his suffering and pain. Meanwhile, he thought it was a good experience in his agitated manic enthusiasm. He wanted to make "our video"! So I owed that video to him and I had to work quite hard to get myself ready to return to it and do it. But I needed to do it, for myself and for him. And then Pato invites me to the Mpowerment group, and this is just what I need: to be immersed in AIDS again and to do the work. I go, and it is great.

TED: The Mpowerment youth are living the legacy and inheritances of AIDS.

ALEX: That's how I saw it, yes.

TED: And both Pato as the group leader, and you as the person behind the camera, share a lot of prior experience with HIV. It is interesting for me to watch what is not there on the screen, but must have been in place for the images to even exist. You are both generous, making space for them and yourselves to all be there. And the youth do what they do, say what they want and need to say, sometimes incorrect, sometimes stigmatizing, always insightful.

ALEX: Well, remember, I edited the piece from hours of footage. They said lots of things, and I selected these takes. The things they say that are beautiful, and those that make me sad, then and now. And I can't help feeling . . . I don't know, frustrated, or confused, or . . . I guess just beaten down. Only ten years after AIDS Crisis Culture, they have lost much of the vocabulary (and associated analysis and action) my generation of AIDS activists worked so hard to build: around community, self-empowerment, and self-love in the face of HIV; around homophobia, racism, and other forms of systemic attack. In the tape, you can hear how they self-blame for HIV, or even for their gayness. How they self-destruct or even self-harm. Because they somehow lack words to understand this as the racist, homophobic, AIDS-phobia that it is, they blame themselves.

147

TED: A direct impact of silence, that loss. When I think about all the conversations not had within the Second Silence, I get very sad. It was like a decade of possibility or more was stolen from us.

ALEX: I make that an overt theme of the piece. I record the kids talking about the issues that are live for them and also ask them to consider issues that are important to me: the forgetting of AIDS, the relevance (or lack thereof) of the stories of people who died to their generation. At some point I ask them, "Does it matter to you, these stories of gay white men, who you would never have met, even if they had lived?" and "What about the history of AIDS activism?" I use their answers under images of Jim on the beach. The original footage plays in real time for the entirety of the art video that I made from and about it.

TED: And if I can interject, this is a moment I love because you are really making a cacophony of silences here.

ALEX: Are you talking about how, along with the MPowerment footage, I also use audio tape of the phone conversations I recorded with lesbian feminist AIDS activists who I knew in the 1980s in New York, people I had made work with previously and with whom I discuss the fact that we don't talk about AIDS together anymore? If so, it is interesting that you say silences instead of voices.

TED: Yes. I love this mix. If we are saying that silence is a process, a pairing, a twinning that is not about absence, when I hear them speaking, I hear their relationship to what they were feeling and thinking about within the Second Silence. They are sharing their silences. I think it is a strong part of your video.

ALEX: Thanks. We talk about remembering and not remembering AIDS. We talk about where it's gone. We talk about the silence. About why we do and do not talk about AIDS and about what we have made, even so, before and since. I interviewed Ellen, as well as Alisa Lebow, Juanita Mohammed Szczepanski, and Sarah Schulman. Their voices also play under Jim. And a few times, when my interviewees recall a video from the past, I cut to it, blended on top of the unrolling images of Jim on the beach. There are really powerful images of Essex Hemphill and Marlon Riggs that join him on the tape. My friends and I remember them—and then the video cuts to their images—how they made such amazing art: poetry, video, dance, in the Black gay community, and how they died even so.

148

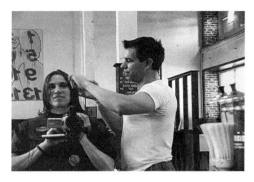

9.6 Michael cutting Alex's hair. Still from *Video Remains*.

TED: This witnessing of a few of the many losses of AIDS is hard. But I take sustenance from your friends holding on to their memories, just as does the video. Like you, the women you interview lived on and they are witnesses. They tell you that they don't often find the time or space to talk about the weight of AIDS on their everyday lives, and that the conversation, while sad, is necessary.

ALEX: That's what the video's doing and modeling: creating a space for a collective, supported return to this pain and quiet, embedded in community and its loss, and what video has to do and can do about this.

TED: They say that they had to move on.

ALEX: This is the Second Silence in action: none of us were speaking, we were remembering in private (or repressing), there was little to no public conversation. There were so many reasons for this, and so many more to break out of this paralysis and quiet (the ongoing needs of the youth I met being primary; getting out of our own isolation, important as well).

TED: And then there is the last element of the video . . .

ALEX: I think you are talking about the interview I shot with the stylist who cut my hair, Michael, who I chanced upon in a Silver Lake salon. He was cutting my hair and he just starts talking to me about stuff: shooting the shit. And the next thing you know, we're talking about something so unexpected and far away—AIDS in New York City; our shared AIDS Crisis Culture—and he's telling me all these stories of people he had lost. This is the real experience that actually happened at a haircut, before I restaged the encounter and shot video of it. In both instances, we acknowledge how necessary and moving it feels to be having that conversation (again, after so many years),

149

that New York conversation, in Los Angeles. To have a conversation about AIDS, and to have a conversation with someone who also lost people about those we've lost. We hadn't been doing it. So I shot this for the tape, and cut him in because he's someone else through whom AIDS had come alive for me again. I restaged that conversation, but it's real. He brings to life many people that had been important to him who died, and what it feels like to live among people who were dying, only then to carry them forward. He does that as part of his professional practice while cutting hair and with other clients, and he modeled it for my camera so that I could use it in the video.

TED: Now I understand why you shot him in the mirror. It is another example of twinning. Together you are Silence +.

ALEX: How sweet. How intense. I needed a role model, and an ally, and someone to prop me up. Michael entered my life and had a conversation with me when I wasn't having conversations, when I was in my silence. It was a powerful moment of coming up against and getting out of silence, and I wouldn't or couldn't deny him. He's a great storyteller. And then he tells those same real and sad stories for my tape. I only shot it once. It's not staged, really. It's just—he's doing what he does, what he has to do.

And to be technical for a second, this is the one other long take in the video. And it is about witnessing, trauma, and memory—as was the first hour of footage of Jim on the beach. But as a part of my feminist documentary practice, I carefully put myself with Michael in this frame. While the scene is mostly Michael speaking in close-up, we are together holding visual space for a shared guilt and anguish and responsibility (and not just ours but that of our generation of survivors). I try for that footage to be ennobling for Michael, much as Jim had wanted his to be. But because I know that that failed for Jim, I am aware that Michael and I both might also be failed by the camera or maybe even each other. That's one reason I also shoot the young people. So many questions of failure are live in the video. Did my generation fail them? Are they failing us? I blend their images with Jim's on the beach to show there is this connection, as well as many possible misses, and also mutual responsibilities.

So I put Michael into the tape because, like Pato and the youth and women, he's another person who allowed AIDS to come alive for me again, and with whom I was healing by talking about it. I say, "I'm ready." I'm ready to deal with my dead tape of a dead friend. This is also a way of saying that I am ready to deal with a live AIDS, and ready for AIDS to deal with me. Again.

TED: AIDS is not a solo experience, yet the Second Silence, as is true for the First, was built upon disconnect. The ongoing if disparate expressions in the Second Silence went largely unconnected. Activities of great import were released to end up falling into a void. Maybe burst with clarity but igniting nothing more. In the Second Silence, the lack of space afforded AIDS in public meant that our responses never became organized, catalyzed, or recognized.

ALEX: But Ted, I think what both of our projects during the Second Silence show us is that while there is an administrative and systemic violence that came as a result of the lack of cultural conversation, there was and are other human costs to the Second Silence. The person I loved the most in the world died when we were both young. I felt and feel a responsibility to stay true to everything I owe him. If he was alive today, I would be staying true in all the ways I do to my friends now. We would have coffee. I would make art with him. I don't know. He'd be part of my family. I'd visit him wherever he now lived. I'd call him when I needed advice or affirmation. We'd be writing a book or play about AIDS. I don't know where he'd be. He is dead, and so I can't do or know any of those things. And he's been dead now for a very long time and now I'm middle-aged. And in my whole life, even so, even today, he's one of the most important people I have, and in some ways he has become the *most* important, because he died. I feel utterly responsible to stay true to him, to all of the hims. He's mine, but there were and are thousands, tens of thousands, millions of those human beings for whom someone is staying true. And all of that is made even harder because he actually died in anguish and pain, and then, a few years later, I was living in California in the flowers. That just felt terrible. And to be really clear here, at the time, I feel guilty and ashamed that I wasn't strong enough.

TED: You keep saying that and I keep on thinking I understand you, but maybe I don't. What do you mean, strong enough for what?

ALEX: To keep doing it.

TED: Keep doing what?

ALEX: Being an activist. Not just remembering . . . fighting.

TED: Because that's a part of him that you want to be true to?

ALEX: No. He wasn't an activist, really. Jim was an artist, and a bon vivant, and a mess, and a young man not yet grown really. I want to be strong enough

151

to be true to him by being an AIDS activist. By keeping the fight alive. Keeping our attention on AIDS. Allowing people to remember that AIDS happened and is happening. But thinking this through here, I am not sure Jim and his memory are the only motivating factors in my work. That seems too instrumentalizing, especially when it comes to *Video Remains*. I really don't know if I have words to describe the role Jim plays in me, in my life since he died, or in my AIDS work: just that he is ever-present and I do the work for him and from him. And so when I met Pato, I saw an opportunity to move from guilt to action.

TED: Do you think that people have to know who Jim is to you to understand the video?

ALEX: Yes and no. I think that people from that time will know exactly the space that Jim takes up in my life and the world, because almost everyone still doing AIDS work from our generation has their own Jim. Anyone who has lost someone to HIV is communicating with the dead as they also find strength from their new friends who are alive. People bring to the video their own constellation of experiences and friends, and their own losses and joy: their lens through which to view, feel—and absorb! So while someone may have a more specific view of the video if they are given my biography or if they "know more about Jim," I hope that you can have no access to the real me, or Jim, or anyone in that video and still walk away with a sense of what is going on in the Silence.

TED: What I like about what you are saying is that the video is about Jim, of course, but it is also about you and him, and the version of your friendship that others will witness, recognize, understand.

ALEX: Yes, and for people to link all that to HIV. Maybe the best way to explain who he is to me today is to remind you of what I said in the oral history we did together for the Smithsonian.[3] I named Jim as my "best enabler," and that feels the most right. Which is different from motivation. I am not trying to make him into a proud warrior or to avenge his death. Rather: he saw something in me, and I saw something in him, and together we made the world more possible for what we needed and wanted to be as humans, if only for a short time. And so the work I am doing now is and will always be indebted to that power we had and made together and which I must now shoulder alone (which is impossible, by definition). How he helped me to become a better person, or even just the grown-up I am. I could never have done AIDS work the way I have without our friendship. Even with the friend-

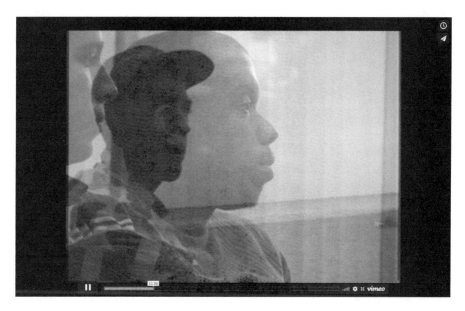

9.7 Jim caught in the blur. Still from *Video Remains*.

ship that you and I now have in this work, Ted, I lean on Jim. Does that make sense?

TED: Sure. And also, it doesn't need to make sense.

ALEX: Exactly. As Jim helped me see, things can be ridiculous, and too much, and beyond comprehension at first, and there is some value in that—letting the world swirl in its capacious confusion. We need each other to make sense of the world. In this sense, a person is at a disadvantage if you think you can understand something all by yourself!

TED: That idea of needing each other is one of the most important parts of the video, *non*?

ALEX: Oh, yes. Yes. I needed Jim. Jim needed me. And I needed Juanita, Sarah, Alisa, and Ellen, and they needed me, at least then. And then again years later when I made the video. You hear it. In the phone conversations that's actually what I'm talking to the other women about because none of us are doing it anymore: being in a world defined by AIDS. They're all like, "I can't believe you're remembering to do that!" Everyone says that: "Thank you so much for making me think about it."

TED: Wait, so that makes me curious, or maybe sensitive to this notion of guilt that you brought up earlier. Is it something you are dealing with every morning, or is it something that catches you by surprise? Is it both? Is it something else?

ALEX: I think it's a nagging. Do you know how the people that you love who have died talk to you?

TED: Yes.

ALEX: It's like that. But he's not a grandparent. He's not an old person. He's like my other half. A young half. And he died. Jim was silenced by AIDS and stuck in the year and time and epoch in which he suffered and died. But what he means to me, and how he speaks to me changes as I live on, and as AIDS changes.

TED: So he's communicating and his life is communicating to you during this period?

ALEX: Yes, he is: during that period, and this one, too. When I try my best to honor, listen to the Jim who is in and with me, this is a fundamental act of salvaging the past, for me. Remembering Jim, bringing him into the present, where he is useful to me and perhaps others, too. Which is why I turn him into art for me and for others. But that is not the only thing that is going on. Do you know how you feel guilty if you're not working against Trump every minute? Do you know what I'm talking about?

TED: Sure.

ALEX: That's what it felt like then. There's this thing. I know it's there. It's inside of me. Why aren't I working on it every minute? That guilt is very real.

TED: Can we pivot for a second?

ALEX: Sure.

TED: Do you think that *Video Remains* is the beginning of the end of the Second Silence?

ALEX: *Video Remains* is a breaking-the-silence video. It gave permission to a still-quieted audience to begin to talk again about AIDS. That's initially how it was received: with grief and conversation opening out into the room. People talking about what it's like to be around someone who's dying who hadn't said that aloud. That's really what people want to talk about when they see that video. And the silence.

154

TED: Say more.

ALEX: *Video Remains* names that AIDS is still very active—not just a thing of the past that we are mourning—alive in us as grief, but also as the HIV in people's bodies and the HIV people will or will not acquire in the future. It is alive for the boys in MPowerment whose futures are still very much before them. It is at once a Silence and Revisitation video. In silence it uses the past to release me from my slumber and enter the present. Does that answer your question?

TED: Maybe. I don't know. Can I talk about myself again?

ALEX: Sure.

TED: Okay, so I ended up doing an exhibition of my Polaroids at a nightclub in Edmonton. The whole thing was really beautiful. HIV Edmonton even paid to have a zine made. My friend Q. C., who at that time worked at HIV Edmonton, wrote a beautiful line in the introduction: "AIDS is not over, but we don't need to be afraid anymore. Instead, we should be standing naked and queer before the world shouting 'This is my body. Witness me! . . . It's time to stand strong in our sexualities. It's time to make love again courageously through the night. Let us heal our wounds and love our scars. Let us embrace ourselves and each other.'"[4]

But in the end, I am not sure if we did anything to make a dent in the Second Silence, even locally. I think the project made an impact within the lives of the people it touched, but I know that the project exists firmly within the Second Silence because it didn't spark other things when it comes to HIV/AIDS. It was written about on a blog by one of my friends, and she got it, but that was kinda it. Even some members of the HIV Edmonton community, amid their support, couldn't fully grasp or get behind what I was doing. All of us to some degree thought that silence was going to be the permanent state of AIDS. We saw it as being as big of a hurdle as the virus itself. Silence=AIDS.

I would say that *Video Remains*, because of who you included, how it got made, and how it was received, had a different impact than anything I was doing. Something more than sparks were made from it, small fires started to burn.

ALEX: Maybe that specific project of yours did not break the silence in your communities as you wished it may have by inspiring new work and larger actions elsewhere. But I see it, and your other artwork, and your community work, as your AIDS work in Silence. And that, along with all the other hopeful, angry, ongoing Second Silence practices, was part of what eventually broke the larger silence because you and others just kept starting fires, more and more of them, and then doing the harder work of keeping them all aflame, and making connections between them.

TED: But maybe we need to move away from the fire metaphor. Maybe it is better to see how our efforts were less about starting flames, and more about cracking through the silence, noticing that silence is never total (unless you are dead), and that it is speckled and colored and live with possibility waiting to happen.

ALEX: Silence and Ending-Silence are twinned, connected. I'm not sure when the silence ended, or if it ended. Maybe in some communities it is still rolling, swirling, opening up, and then clouding over. What I do know is that for me, for you, and most likely for people reading this book, the Second Silence is over.

TED: Which is not to say that there are not still more silences within the Times of AIDS—

ALEX: But that the very muchness that had been siloed is now better networked.

TED: Living within silence means that you can have a group of people fighting for their lives in the most savvy, urgent, and profound ways, making as much noise as they can, while simultaneously another group of people, those with ignorance and malice, can ignore, not reach out, or factor in those people while making choices that will cause death, all because there is not a spark, or a broadcast, or a platform. So I reiterate, Silence is not absence.

ALEX: Only in its most thorough state, what we might call *fully realized silence*, is it completely devitalizing, an actual abyss of darkness that does and is nothing. But Silence + is what was experienced, practiced, and lived through for those of us who didn't die. We have come to understand through our many conversations about silence—and also our many false starts—that we are always talking about Silence +.

TED: Which makes me want to return to the Silence = Death from yet another, final vantage. The poster. The crew who made it (the Silence=Death project) are very specific that it was a form of propaganda made to look like there was a large organized response to AIDS, even if there wasn't.

ALEX: They named and pictured a response into being!

TED: Yes. They communicated a sign of competence to the general public. But also, and maybe more importantly, they communicated a vision of community and a movement to others impacted by HIV who were feeling overwhelmed and isolated. This was needed because of the impacts of Reagan's and other's silence.

ALEX: I remember seeing those signs everywhere in downtown New York City (I went to the second ACT UP demo and then a meeting shortly thereafter because of them). A sort of beacon that drew us together out of the First Silence.

TED: People were having their own individual experiences with death and illness, as well as with activism and care, but because of the first cover of silence, it was hard to connect these responses or experiences. The poster cut through the silence and created a means to connect the disparate sounds of pain, love, action, and people.

ALEX: Making art about silence is hard.

TED: And making art about silence is part of what we all need to move into action.

ALEX: Conversation between peers, movements, artists, and within and across communities builds power. Cultural objects initiate, record, and move forward conversation. Conversation can locate, love, and build again from such objects or people with keen attention to what people need and do now. Shall we try that next?

+ VIDEO

9 SILENCE + VIDEO

1 SILENCE + YOU

Consider a time when someone could see you more clearly than you could see yourself. How could you represent what they saw?

2 SILENCE + OTHERS

Use what you came up with to begin a conversation about the experience of being seen. Can you make something that represents this in a medium of your choice to share? Consider how or if you could record this conversation.

3 SILENCE + THE WORLD

Like *Video Remains,* here are four AIDS activist videos that we identify as feminist practices of care:

- *We Care: A Video for Care Providers of People Affected by AIDS.* The Women's AIDS Video Enterprise, 1990.
- *Two Men and a Baby.* Juanita Mohammed (Szczepanski), 1997.
- *Shatzi Is Dying.* Jean Carlomusto, 2000.
- *The Whole World Is Watching.* J Triangular, 2019.

10 SILENCE + UNDETECTABILITY

ALEX: The Second Silence lingered like a low hanging cloud for much longer than any of us wanted. When things finally begin to pierce this, what follows was felt as curious, invigorating, and intense. Cultural activities or objects bring people together after being siloed, quiet, or disengaged: to see new work, but also to talk about the Revisitation itself.

TED: The period that we call the AIDS Crisis Revisitation begins around 2008. It heralds possibilities that quickly yield what will grow into a large body of new AIDS cultural production. As we experienced—and continue to experience—this outpouring of cultural *returns*, we understand that these works have much in common. But most critically for us, they are built first and foremost from a backward look at the death and illness, compassion and dignity, as well as the urgent and often effective community responses that were related to HIV . . . *as it was experienced in the past.*

ALEX: This is why we call it the Revisitation.

TED: These works cull from and curate footage, photos, memories, art, and ephemera from the First Silence and AIDS Crisis Culture. Their revisited content comes from personal collections as well as individual and institutional archives and museums (such as the New York Public Library and the Fales Library & Special Collections, NYU, the Whitney, the Tate), as well as previous art works and documentaries.

ALEX: This inspired what would become our interest in archives, histories, and salvage: that is, trying to figure out who saved these things that were being revisited, how, for whom, and how this could be done again, if differently, via inclusion and conversation.

TED: Indeed. Through our conversation about all this work, which itself became part of the Revisitation and was joined and amplified by that of many of our peers, we learned that the earliest work in the Revisitation relied heavily on footage of pre-gentrified urban centers populated by passionate twenty-somethings fighting for their lives. This conjured up memories and trauma for some, nostalgia for those who were not alive at the time and some who were, and a hope for others about a possible return to such an engaged moment (without all the loss).

ALEX: It is an impressive movement of media, art, and culture that attempts to look back, find, historicize, learn, and feel from what happened in the previous Times of AIDS. But in much of this work, its pastness also makes it ring as if AIDS is something that is over. By making use of a clarity and distance only available through the retrospective and the already-completed, an end-stop is set.

TED: We developed most of our theories and practices by spending time with Revisitation projects, with each other, in our communities.

ALEX: Why don't we honor some of the earliest work that propelled us out of silence?

TED: Some examples of the early and much discussed Revisitation work are the films *We Were Here* (David Weissman and Bill Weber, 2011), *United in Anger* (Jim Hubbard, 2012), or the art project turned short film *Last Address* (Ira Sachs, 2010). Over the past ten or so years there have been scores of other films, as remarkable in their number as was the silence that preceded their creation (see Timeline 3).

ALEX: There were a great many museum exhibitions like *Why We Fight: Remembering AIDS Activism* (New York Public Library, 2013); retrospectives like those about Gran Fury (80WSE, NYU 2012), General Idea (Musée d'Art Moderne, 2011), and Frank Moore (Grey Art Gallery, NYU, 2012); and smaller gallery shows, such as the remount of Rosalind Solomon's exhibition, *Portraits in the Time of AIDS*, 1988 (Bruce Silverstein Gallery, 2013), just to name a few.

160

TED: Nonfiction books emerged, such as *Fire in The Belly: The Life and Times of David Wojnarowicz*, by Cynthia Carr (2012). And there were fictional backward glances like *Christadora* by Tim Murphy (2016) or *The Great Believers* by Rebecca Makkai (2018).

ALEX: During this period there was a reemergence of AIDS activism through new collectives (such as QUEEROCRACY) and the revitalization of preexisting groups (AIDS ACTION NOW in Toronto, and ACT UP in New York and San Francisco). While these groups were focused on AIDS of the present, their formation, or reformation as it were, allowed a new generation of younger activists to begin from a base inspired by or rooted in the AIDS activism of the past. They were hoping to build upon previous work, connections, community, representation, and visuals.

TED: There was a revival of *The Normal Heart* on Broadway and then a remake on HBO, as well as less categorizable work such as Kirk Read's reading series and collective from 2012, *The Biggest Quake* (featuring Mark Abramson, Justin Chin, Brontez Purnell, Carol Queen, Julia Serano, K. M. Soehnlein, and Ed Wolf), which brought together writers creating new work about the past and the present of AIDS; the Smithsonian's 2018 Visual Artists and AIDS oral history project, which interviewed artists and others involved in the art world from the 1980s and 1990s impacted by HIV (including my oral history of you, from which we learned a great deal that would inform this process); Danspace's multiplatform project "Platform 2016: Lost and Found," curated by Ishmael Houston-Jones and Will Rawls, which took a generous look at the legacy of AIDS within the dance and performance world of New York; and so on.

ALEX: We can see the Revisitation as a response, a reaction, a reengagement with the Second Silence. A (re)turn toward AIDS, if you will, just as Douglas Crimp had said we turned away in 1981.

TED: Within the cultural landscape, the Revisitation made AIDS visible again—

ALEX: At least initially for (and about) gay white men: a devastated and damaged community, our friends and brothers and allies, many of whom for the first time in the cultural and physical life of AIDS were seeing and often enjoying ongoing and improving health. Revisitation is a Silence Recovering Project.

TED: So true. That's really clarifying. And as we will document soon, we are particularly interested in learning about how these high-profile works of visibility created conversation where there had only recently been silence, conversation in communities and between isolated individuals all hungry to engage about AIDS given years of famine: in intended communities, between

161

communities, and within communities who found these works valuable in their focus on AIDS, or memory, trauma, history, or personal archives. But there were still many people who needed to see their own stories and voices added to this growing historical and personal reckoning.

ALEX: The diverse, exciting, and generative conversations that were inspired by works of the AIDS Crisis Revisitation—including those of criticism, reaction, embellishment, addition, soul-searching, discord, love, and memorial—shape and reshape the move from silence, one which had been particularly stuck because during the Second Silence the meds had made HIV itself undetectable!

TED: Ah! Alex, the word we have been so careful not to engage until now. We have felt so conflicted about when best to use that word in its many valences. Undetectable is a big part of what we have been talking about, without using the word . . .

ALEX: Or, shall we say, "silenced" . . . *by us.*

TED: AIDS went undetectable within the Second Silence.

ALEX: And then again, many people who are undetectable have chosen to stay undetectable, even during the Revisitation. AIDS did not go away, it did not disappear, it was and is still present, but for many it went largely unseen through first a medical, and then a cultural, personal, and/or political project of knowing but not seeing and therefore forgetting, displacing, or not saying.

TED: We could have easily used the word "undetectable" when discussing the Second Silence, but I silenced it between us until now because in recent years it has come to refer to something very specific within the world of HIV: a new status for people living with HIV.

ALEX: In 2017, the Prevention Access Campaign (PAC) launched the U = U slogan, Undetectable = Untransmittable, a catchy, helpful, and meaningful way to educate people that if you are living with HIV and are on a medical treatment plan that works for you, then the virus can be suppressed so much so that it becomes *undetectable,* meaning that antibodies are not findable or measurable in your blood and so the virus is also untransmittable.

TED: As a slogan, U = U seemed to catch on overnight. This was primarily through the tenacity of the PAC, specifically Bruce Richman, the founding executive director.[1] Within months and years, the CDC, UNAIDS, and others

162

were endorsing U = U, after years of being relatively quiet about the science behind the slogan that had been long known.

ALEX: Yet another silence that opened into language and detection, albeit about undetectability. So here we have this perfect word to describe a cultural experience that has also become a powerful way for people to describe their virus, and themselves.

TED: Totally. "I am undetectable" is a term people living with HIV use, be it casually with friends, on hook-up apps, or as a form of activism. Housing Works put out a comic called "The Undetectables," which positioned people living with HIV who have reduced their viral load as superheroes.[2]

ALEX: Which is not without its concerns.

TED: One of the social side effects of U = U is the pressure people living with HIV may feel to get to undetectable, which is not easy or even possible for everyone due to issues of drug access, drug efficacy within some bodies, and systemic issues of adherence—which fall along racial and class lines.

ALEX: Like everything within AIDS history and culture, breaks, cracks, and differences are bound by race, class, location, sexuality, and access to care.

TED: People with greater stability, and more access to and trust in care, are more likely to be able to take their meds and become undetectable than those who have insecure housing, medical providers that don't listen to them, or hurdles in securing the calories needed to take medications.

ALEX: So one of the most curious conditions of the Revisitation, for us, was how U came to equal V. Undetectability = Visibility. This came through the Revisitation, its backward look. The past, which was a time before U, somehow gave us permission we needed to see and be seen again. As you said, the information behind U = U is not new. What is new (again) is that we can see AIDS anyway, now.

TED: Alex! That is so smart. Not to mansplain, but to gush for a minute: I love how in your formulation of U = V you create a Second Silence straddling mashup that identifies the equation as an enduring form of AIDS representation highlighting the connections between survival, representation, and public education. You bring together the explicit message of Silence = Death and the implicit message of U = U to illustrate the fact that visibility matters on a fundamental level to the livelihood of people living with HIV.

163

ALEX: But there is also an inherent contradiction that I am interested in pointing out around how only upon viral suppression was and is AIDS again able to reenter the mass social discourse.

TED: It reminds us that in our thinking, each shift in an AIDS representational epoch is coupled with another change within treatment or policy. The First Silence is a result of (what we would come to call) HIV being recognized at all; AIDS Crisis Culture comes amid introduction of AZT and early iterations of HIV tests, and lasts until the release of life-saving medication, which makes possible the many kinds of withdrawals of the Second Silence, broken only by Revisitation, which flourishes alongside and maybe because of U = U and the introduction of PrEP.

ALEX: But like everything about AIDS, changes are connected to but are never only about a medical shift. To be specific for a second, the Revisitation begins when better health (for those lucky enough to have it) is experienced through time and space: enough distance from the plague years and its death, pain, and drama so that people affected by HIV could begin to heal personally and communally from trauma (or were ready to try). So to zoom out again, I get the calendar of cultural shifts and advancements that you are laying out here. I am interested in thinking about this idea that the Revisitation and U = U are one and the same moment.

TED: I think the mood of the time dictates the shifts to come, and maybe vice versa. I am starting to consider questions around the social and material conditions that make looking back at history possible. You begin to answer this when you remind us that the Revisitation occurs after some people have had enough time away from the heady, public, and shared trauma of AIDS in the 1980s and 1990. This notion of space is important because, as we know, the knowledge of U = U is as old as the Second Silence, which is to say as old as HAART. It is the basis of treatment as prevention, a way of thinking that emerged from the 1996 breakthrough. The thinking was if systems can be put in place to treat, that is to say suppress, the virus in people living with HIV, then we are caring for people with the virus and preventing transmission—which has not happened as of yet.

ALEX: But let's back up. Why has it taken so long for the content of U = U to become common knowledge? How in a very short amount of time, and after such a long time, did the amount of people that understood the impact of being on treatment as it relates to transmission go from very low to very high?

TED: Well, this is where I think our theories about the pulse of AIDS via culture can be helpful. Activist Sean Strub has suggested that the best thing to come out of the First Silence was poz empowerment.[3] I agree, when it comes to the Second Silence, I think poz empowerment was one of the biggest casualties.

ALEX: How do you figure?

TED: If in the First Silence people living with HIV were brought together to fight for their lives out of dire urgency and necessity, in the Second Silence that togetherness was broken apart. For people living with the virus within the Second Silence, HIV went from a robust and public conversation to one primarily held in private with medical providers. This reduced the cultural and political power that people living with HIV had built up over time.

ALEX: Which means the focus went from building power among impacted people, to services for them and the medical model. The Second Silence resulted in a shift, as you often say, from AIDS being a public concern to a private affair.

TED: Exactly, and within the medical model, people living with HIV still found ways to make real and meaningful contributions, often advocating for changes within the systems that had been set up to serve them. This resulted in the creation of Client Advisory Boards (CABS), people living with HIV speaking truth to power when it came to how ASOs should be run. This was and is important work, but one drawback of the CAB format is that it ensures that "clients" are speaking to and about management, and less with and about each other.

ALEX: It is not true that in silence there are *no* conversations being had nor stories being told. Are you saying in silence we tell no stories?

TED: On the contrary, in silence we tell a lot of stories, to ourselves and for ourselves. And this is where the danger lies. Part of what we are modeling here through our practices of intentional conversation is that more voices = different information. In dialogue we learn new things, consider things we may have otherwise missed, and empathy becomes part of our process. But in silence, conversation is siloed. That is what I meant earlier when I said there was no exchange. In silence, communication is largely one-way and underheard, or at the very least underengaged. It lacks pushback, additions, modulations. The violence of silence is that it hampers the flow of ideas, the sharing of experiences.

+ UNDETECTABILITY

ALEX: Within the Second Silence I was isolated from AIDS, in part because I could be. I am not living with HIV. So intentional or not, I was able to walk away. If the virus is in you, and you have a fidelity to treatment, how isolated are you? We do know that many people feel less isolated because of HIV.

TED: A lot of stories were being told within the Second Silence, especially about science and medicine and how they relate to bodies, wellness, illness, culture, and death. But these stories were not finding their way into the larger cultural conversations as they once had, and we are saying here, that was a problem.

ALEX: What is interesting is how U = U, for better or worse, establishes people living with HIV as safe citizens, as people taking care of their illness.

TED: That is interesting. I think you are right. In a way, by establishing the role of the medical model in people's lives, which is implicit within U = U, people living with HIV are granted a new visibility. So for me, the questions are, at what cost, and on whose terms?

ALEX: And again, for better or worse, this impacts the circulation of voices, who is heard, what gets repeated, what ideas drag forward. And then, in moments of peak visibility it is important to remember that conversation can be both progressive and regressive, antagonistic and supportive, and a lot of the work is actually trying to reconcile competing viewpoints and ideologies.

TED: Ethical concerns aside, I am excited about a greater integration into the cultural space of people living with HIV outside of the waiting room. I think part of a healthy culture (about well-being) occurs within different "town squares," if you will, where ideas can be discussed, explored, uncovered, and debated.

ALEX: "The commons" where people talk and listen and can also be liked, loved, made love to, taken care of. I think we are here getting into ideas of trust and community, to which I am adding and celebrating the body. Obviously, some people will have a strong bond with their medical team and will be able to have open and frank discussions with them, while at the same time many of us can't say how we truly feel around our family and friends.

TED: That is the cruelty of the Second Silence. It stopped the flow of conversation, which is a means of blocking power.

ALEX: Until the Revisitation.

166

TED: Which has brought people together. The wide circulation and discourse of the Revisitation acts like a light that we as moths are drawn to.

ALEX: So content and community can work together in the same way we suggest silence and isolation have been so easily aligned.

TED: We are saying that ideas of progress and visibility are also intertwined in the story of HIV.

167

10 SILENCE + UNDETECTABILITY

1 SILENCE + YOU

What is something that people don't see about you and HIV? Represent it.

2 SILENCE + OTHERS

Do you want to share what you made with another? Can you?

3 SILENCE + THE WORLD

Here are two texts about undetectability:

- Nathan Lee. "Becoming-Undetectable." *e-flux Journal*, no. 44 (April 2013). https://www.e-flux.com/journal/44/60170/becoming -undetectable/.

- Thomas Cardamone and Ben Tuttle. *The Undetectables*. New York: Housing Works, 2014–2016. https://liveundetectable.org /comics.

11 SILENCE + CONVERSATION

TED: Our first chapters in this part revealed that even as the Revisitation was ramping up around us, we both still felt isolated. I didn't need the Revisitation to name that for me. What I did need was help to see that silence needn't be the default when it came to AIDS. If we understand that a critical aspect of the Second Silence is that it kept people apart, then the Revisitation can be understood as the first period of time, in a long time, that brings people together, into connection, albeit through the past of AIDS.

ALEX: And the past is just the thing to break people out of silence for many reasons, which is why the Revisitation has been such a fruitful, exciting, and developing period within the history we are telling.

TED: That is what we hoped to establish by telling our own stories. We are just two of so many people who had not forgotten about AIDS, who did not think it was over, and were in fact doing what we could to keep the conversation going all through the long Silence.

ALEX: Only we were doing so in almost complete isolation. When did you first start to see the Revisitation in your life? When did you start to feel you were speaking and listening to and with a crowd?

TED: 2010: when David Wojnarowicz's video *Fire in My Belly* was censored as part of the exhibition *Hide/Seek: Difference and Desire in American Portraiture* at the National Portrait Gallery in Washington, DC. Around the world, artists

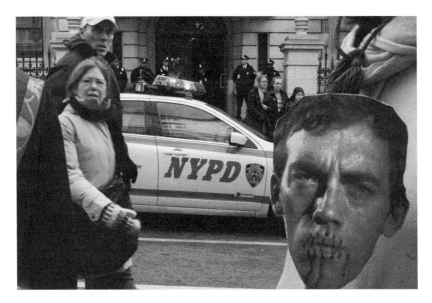

11.1 Hide/Seek protests (2010).

and activists, along with galleries, museums, and other art organizations, responded by screening the video for free and sharing it widely online, hosting public discussions about David's work and career, and organizing protests. In New York there was a march that started at the Metropolitan Museum of Art with people waving placards, chanting, and creating spectacles through their dress and action.

ALEX: I do want to remind you how censorship is the ultimate silence. A good deal of AIDS activism has historically come as a response to this, the most extreme act of silencing.

TED: Maybe that is why people coming together felt so powerful at this time. I was so moved by the conversations that were happening along the march, as well as in the days, months, and years following. It was in these personal connections, bounded and initiated by David—and so also art, culture, and HIV—that people started to talk, share, ask questions, trust, confide, disclose, and soon plot and collaborate as I had longed for, as I had attempted so often to initiate at this scale and intensity during the years before. For me, this protest stands as a day where silence was remembered, used, and ultimately broken so that conversation about AIDS could be rekindled.

ALEX: A few years after that event, the Revisitation worked its magic to bring us together. I was also already thinking about similar things, albeit without your powerful nomenclature, particularly in a set of articles I had recently coauthored with three other scholar/activists about the increasing deluge of AIDS media.[1] Anyone at that time who happened to be writing about HIV/AIDS culture, or making a career in an AIDS-related cultural institutions, wouldn't have been able *not to notice*, wonder, and try to figure out what the fuck was happening with all the content after what felt like such a long drought! The Revisitation was as noticeable, disorienting, shocking, and needing of understanding as had been the Silence. However, in this period, the conversation we all began to have about why it was happening, what it was and wasn't doing, who was doing it and why, simply added to the volume and intensity.

Our brief online interview put you on my radar, and so when I was asked to write about *Dallas Buyers Club* for the film journal *Cineaste*, I reached out to you for a few reasons, not least of which was my desire to do AIDS work again with someone else who seemed smart, curious, and in the know.

TED: And it was through writing about that film that we began together to name, think, and talk about many of the other films and videos—mainstream and alternative and art—that were suddenly entering the cultural landscape, all of which also looked through a backward lens at AIDS, such as *Sex Positive* (Daryl Wein, 2008). *Sex Positive* is important to me because, like the Wojnarowicz protest, it was another early indication in my life that something was changing. In fact, even before the Hide/Seek protests, it was actually my very first clue. I saw the film in 2008 in New York City. I had come to intern for Visual AIDS, under the direction of Executive Director Amy Sadao and Associate Director Nelson Santos. I was so moved by the newness of the film, and what it was doing in public, that I sat across from the theater and wrote about it.

ALEX: "New" to you but old to me in that it was about a past that I had lived through.

TED: Was it old? It was the first time that I had seen a film about AIDS that was intentionally looking back at history from the point of view of someone not "there" and not in the know. *Sex Positive* was made by Daryl Wein, a young straight white man who had no real connection to HIV beyond being alive at that time. He was amazed that his girlfriend lived next door to Richard Berkowitz, who, with Michael Callen, urged gay men to use affection as a

171

form of harm reduction, and condoms to protect themselves from HIV; what would go on to be called "safer sex." In the film, Wein works to communicate the past of AIDS to those who were not there. In so doing, he also provides footage and a sense of memory for those who were around. He considers what the impact of this past is on the present, lingering on the idea that the past of AIDS has been quickly forgotten. There is a painful scene at the end of the film when all these relatively young people are asked if they know who Richard Berkowitz is and all of them are like, "no." It marks how so much information about AIDS is precarious, in danger of being lost. The film (and its director) become the savior (or saver), the link between the largely unknown past and the ongoing but "AIDS-free" present.

ALEX: In the Smithsonian protests and *Sex Positive* we have examples of productive collisions between what came before and the present; the Revisitation is what had to follow the Second Silence with all its tension, intensity, desire, hope, and grief. There needed to be a recalibration. Yes, a reaction to the Silence, but even more. Not only the production of content about AIDS but ideas that move beyond and within communities, connecting them. With a little hindsight, it seems inevitable that another aspect of all this cross-temporal and spatial production was not just connection but also tension, illumination of bias, and something akin to turf wars, such as who has the right to tell whose AIDS story and what stories are right to tell.

TED: Almost as soon as the Revisitation began it became a place of celebration and new learning for some, a place of self-righteousness for others, a place of mourning and remembering for many, and also a battleground within AIDS communities.

ALEX: Early criticism of Revisitation output, including some of our own, centered on the sameness of much of the work's focus—yes, the past of AIDS but also a largely white, middle-class, US-coastal, cis-male, and gay one—which then resulted in myriad conversations within our communities about the politics of representation as this relates, in particular, to the lack of women, Black people, people of color, trans people, communities from rural, south, and middle America and the rest of the world, particularly the global South, given that these communities were and continue to be disproportionately affected by AIDS, as well as other forms of systemic oppression.

172   TED: For example, there's the 2013 exhibition *AIDS in NYC: The First Five Years* at the New York Historical Society, which our friend Hugh Ryan wrote about in his *New York Times* opinion piece, "How to Whitewash a Plague."[2]

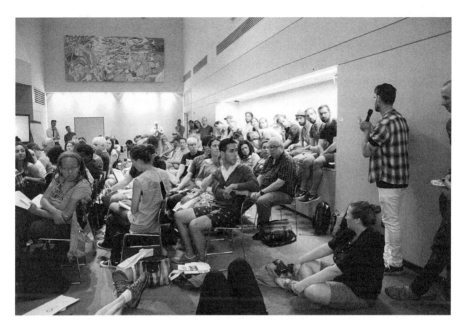

II.2 (re)Presenting AIDS: Culture and Accountability event (2013).

ALEX: He took issue with the ways in which gay men and activists were not part of the museum's telling of the city's AIDS history. Instead, they presented a heroic story of local politics and the medical community.

ALEX: Note the role of heroism in so much of this work, as well. Problem solved through male might!

TED: Hugh was upset not simply about who was being left out, but rather because erasure pointed to a larger problem. He captured this beautifully: "Bad history has consequences. I'm not afraid we will forget AIDS; I am afraid we will remember it and it will mean nothing. If we cannot face the root issue— that we let people die because we did not like them—AIDS will become a blip on our moral radar, and this cycle will repeat every time we connect an unpopular group with something that scares us."[3]

That line was everything to me. I used Hugh's response to galvanize resources at Visual AIDS for something I had wanted to do for a while. I worked with Hugh and others to co-organize a community discussion titled "(re) Presenting AIDS: Culture and Accountability." It took place in 2013 on a hot August night in a packed auditorium at the top of the CUNY Grad Center

173

in Midtown New York. Moderated by ACT UP member Ann Northrup, we organized the event around three core questions:

1 What responsibility do institutions with little to no relationship with those most impacted by HIV/AIDS have when mounting an exhibition related to the ongoing epidemic?
2 As a community of people living with and impacted by HIV, what do we want from cultural institutions when they engage with HIV/AIDS as a topic?
3 As the crisis of AIDS continues, how do we ensure that the stories that need to be shared are told and heard by those who need them the most?

I have fond memories of that event. I felt like people had not only been waiting for years to express what was on their mind to and with others, but that they were hungry for community around AIDS rooted in these very questions of how to talk about not just AIDS in the past but in our shared present. People were really listening. Director Jim Hubbard said something that night that I continue to think about often:

There is a cliché that history is told by the victors, and I feel that in a real sense, people with AIDS and ACT UP were the victors in this. We are the ones who should be telling the story. In a certain way, these institutions are fighting back and what it reminds me of is, one of the questions I get from time to time when I show *United in Anger*, "What about the other side?" And it is a question that really threw me for a while because there is no other side. They were wrong. We have to say that over and over again. Those people who are wrong are going to try and reinvent the story to make themselves look better.

ALEX: I was not there that night. I was still living in LA. But I read the transcript you made available online, pictures and all, and wow![4] For me, meaningful and robust conversations about AIDS, such as the one Visual AIDS and Hugh made possible, are a beautiful bookend to the Second Silence. A room full of people talking about AIDS across differences is what I remember happening frequently in the 1980s and 1990s and is something I am again often a part of today. But during the Second Silence all that had gone away. This was something I missed—and craved—in the early 2000s. I started feeling it as the films came out: bigger films, bigger budgets, and most importantly, larger and increasingly more diverse audiences.

174

TED: Not to backtrack, but this is a good illustration of our difference. While you were missing such conversations, I had waited my whole life to have them.

ALEX: Noted. Can I tell you about one of the conversations that excited me?

TED: Of course!

ALEX: I had my own moment of THE REVISITATION IS HERE! after you circulated my article "Forgetting ACT UP" (2012) and then hosted a reading of it for your PDF Book Club. I was in LA, the club was in New York. I followed along online.

TED: Your essay was so helpful for me during my early days of the Revisitation. It allowed me to respectfully point out the space that ACT UP was taking up in the Revisitation vis-à-vis the films and exhibitions, and the writing and lectures, and how that was contributing to another form of whitewashing beyond the meaningful ways that Hugh had already pointed out. In my experience, as insidious as the erasure of activists during *The First Five Years* art show, was the way that ACT UP had become a stand in for all activism and cultural production within AIDS Crisis Culture. I had not been able to put that into words until I read your line, "When ACT UP is remembered . . . other places, people, and forms of AIDS activism are disremembered."[5] This was helpful because while I don't believe the media is a zero-sum game, I do think the media covering AIDS cannot handle too much nuance. And it seemed almost too much to ask for to have people consider AIDS activism beyond ACT UP.

ALEX: Right, in the drought period of Second Silence any memory or image was a gift. And given the powerful work we did in ACT UP, why not focus attention again on that? We produced amazing actions and art and accomplished important things that were both bold and showy, but also small and meaningful. But in writing that essay, because I now felt we had room again to draw out the richness and diversity of our communities and experiences, I wanted to make space for different registers of AIDS activist pasts to also be remembered and witnessed, and I wanted to provide a platform for people who had their own diverse AIDS activist histories to feel welcome to share even though these had nothing to do with ACT UP.

TED: And it worked! At the event I hosted where we discussed the PDF, people— young, old, and otherwise—spoke about their sense of not feeling that they belonged within the Revisitation because they had not been part of ACT UP or were not interested primarily in ACT UP. Members of ACT UP's Latino Caucus spoke at my reading group about how, even if they were part of ACT UP, there was still a sense of erasure and dislocation in how the history was being told, to date, through film and exhibition.

ALEX: Well, here it is. ACT UP is one of the go-to places for AIDS history, and deservedly so. But importantly, even in the saturation of ACT UP narratives within AIDS recollection, the fullness and complexity within it is often itself left uncaptured. Women, lesbians, people of color, Latin/x, Black, and trans people were part of ACT UP, although we often struggled within the organization to be seen and heard (we addressed this later when we co-curated the art show *Metanoia* with others. Our show included documents of ACT UP's activism concerning women and prison. We devote chapter 14 to this conversation). But as critically, during AIDS Crisis Culture, other groups that focused specifically on women, prison, housing, people of color, drug users, and so on were busy and live across New York City, and around the country and world, doing activism and AIDS work where other needs, services, communities, tactics, and experiences of the epidemic served as their North Star.

TED: And for younger generations: Was there a history for them if the version of ACT UP being shared did not resonate with or include them? Julian DeMayo, who was part of the Forgetting ACT UP discussion, spoke about how early in his master's project about the Latino Caucus of ACT UP, he felt that he needed to make the Latino version of *How to Survive a Plague*. But as he spoke to the members of the caucus, he saw that other strategies—less public, less grandstanding—were what was desired by his community. He was interested in connecting members to each other to share their stories.

ALEX: I thought that was what I was doing, too. So I was pretty surprised when my little essay caused a small tempest in a teapot on the ACT UP NY Facebook alumni page. There were scores of comments to a post someone shared about the event. Most people hadn't gone to the club or read the article. But they responded in anger to the intentionally inflammatory title. One or two were overtly hostile or just weird, but otherwise, it did just what we think is definitive of Revisitation: people began debating, and then listening, learning, and engaging together about the truly hard questions raised by history, memory, forgetting, denying, repressing, self-definition, suffering, health, and difference. The Revisitation was growing and changing as more people were beginning to tell their stories as well as listening to those of others. As hard as it was to be criticized by people who hadn't read my work,

176

and to watch some online flaming that followed, I really was quite happy to see that the article, the event in New York City, as well as on the Facebook thread, was opening up conversation, not shutting it down.

TED: I think about the (re)presenting AIDS and *Forgetting ACT UP* conversations a lot. They were the largest gatherings of concerned and invested people that I had been to, to date, where people who were working in AIDS cultural production and activism came together in one place. Up until then, siloed and unheard, they were now able to share their thoughts, fears, feelings, and questions, and to see they were not alone in this. It was also clear to me that more had to be said and done. So a few months after (re)Presenting AIDS, I organized What You Don't Know About AIDS Could Fill a Museum for a Visual AIDS event at the Brooklyn Museum. It was a smaller affair. I invited Hugh Ryan, along with filmmaker Jean Carlomusto, scholar Tara Burk, and documentary photographer Vincent Cianni. It was moderated by activist and artist Brittney Duck.

ALEX: In reading the transcript of this conversation, I am moved by the intergenerational nature of it all.[6] You have both Jean and Vince who, like myself and James Wentzy, Sarah Schulman, Gregg Bordowitz, Gran Fury, Jim Hubbard, and a small number of others, were artists and activists from the AIDS Crisis Culture generation who never stopped making AIDS-related culture. And they are in conversation with Hugh and Tara, younger people both making a world for themselves and their generation that includes AIDS!

TED: Jean and Vince both spoke to the care that is needed to tend to archives, while in Hugh and Tara we find two people who are very caring within the archive. It was a perfect night, but one that spoke to the one-wayness of AIDS culture at the time: that is, one that is only looking back. It was really hard to move away from the past.

ALEX: But Ted, for so many of us, what you are calling the past was also part of a current discussion, part of us. This is what Jean meant when from the panel she said, "In my current-day practice I do find it important to maintain my archive. That's a part of my current activism, keeping history alive. I see my role now in telling history, to tell people to examine how this history may fit into current discussions about the plague." And it is what I hope you understand about *Video Remains*. "The past" was key to the siloed Second Silence, it was the cat that caught our tongue. The past's losses—of people, community, activism—is what kept us mumbling to ourselves. There is no way that we as individuals, or a culture, could have gone from the Silence to

177

the Revisitation cold turkey. We have too many ghosts, unresolved conversations, and questions. We have unprocessed baggage. We have unresolved trauma. Saying AIDS in public, even with an audience again, was not enough. As it happens, I had an easier time than others because I had made *Video Remains* some years before. I had done some processing, some ramping up to the Revisitation, and in that, I helped others. But hardly anyone had done that within the Silence. While much of the content and tension expressed at the start of the Revisitation was about the politics of representation and inclusion it was also about memory, age, being left out, the dead, and also people's feelings around a sense of duty. This needed to be an intergenerational conversation. That would also become one of our contributions to the Revisitation, that we were talking and writing and publishing and organizing, as a duo, effectively, with compassion and curiosity, and across so much difference.

TED: But these conversations didn't go so smoothly for many of us. I think we have to ask, at what and whose cost was the past being processed, and between whom? These are the hard questions that Vincent Chevalier and Ian Bradley Perrin brought up in their work for PosterVirus, "Your Nostalgia Is Killing Me," in 2013. The poster, shared online and also wheat-pasted in downtown Toronto and other cities, is a beseeching for viewers to consider that there is a price to pay for all this rewarding if useful looking back, especially for people diagnosed after 1996, as well as for the newly seroconverted. Their poster—a digital rendering of a child's bedroom circa the late 1990s, outfitted with the greatest hits from AIDS culture—is a battle cry for the present. They have spoken about how, as two young men living with HIV today, they meet people their own age who have a better sense of AIDS of the past than they do of AIDS now. In an interview I did with them for Visual AIDS, they explained how the poster comes out of both of their experiences of AIDS images from AIDS Crisis Culture being passed around online without attention to either their original context or respect for the present, and an awareness around how the past can foreclose any conversation around the present, what it is to live with HIV or AIDS today, or what HIV/AIDS means today.[7]

ALEX: Like so much, or maybe all material on the internet!

TED: While we can never know who someone's audience is online, my guess is that most of the AIDS Tumblr-related content that Vincent and Ian were seeing was more about virtue-signaling than intentional education or real, thick engagement.

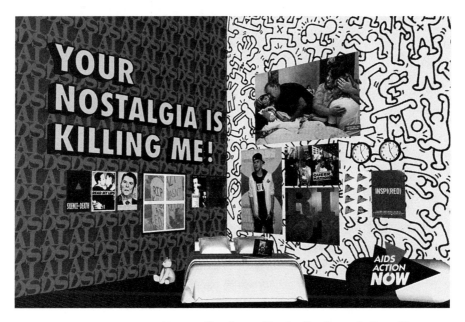

11.3 Vincent Chevalier and Ian Bradley Perrin for PosterVirus, 2013.

ALEX: This is why for me, no matter how rich the internet can be as a tool in our AIDS work, nothing beats being in a room together when possible. AIDS taught me that, and in AIDS I try to keep teaching that.

TED: When they say, "Your nostalgia is killing me," they mean it! All of the cultural fetishization of the past of AIDS that we've been discussing so far (across the ecosystem of AIDS representation) made it almost impossible for people to attend to, let alone conceive of, HIV in the now. That in turn made it harder for people to consider what needs to be done today in response to the ongoing crisis. But as the poster circulated online, some vocal long-term members of ACT UP took offense, feeling as though they were being personally attacked. I was shocked by the ways some of the ACT UP alumni members were unwilling to support young people as they fought for their right to be seen within the context of their own HIV experiences. And so, still at Visual AIDS at the time, we worked with the New York Public Library to host a public discussion about the poster, nostalgia, and AIDS, resulting in yet another intense dialogue, definitive of this moment in the Revisitation, around the various experiences of AIDS that were happening at that moment, simultaneously.

179

ALEX: The past and present can comingle, with care, even and perhaps because there will be a spark. I think when we pause and reflect, we can understand why some long-term survivors and activists felt attacked, just as we can see the validity of the claims of younger people with HIV. There's room in the conversation for all these temporalities, experiences of HIV, and for connections, contradictions, and criticism. What was said, and what did you do to care for your audience?

TED: A lot of things, including artist Kia LaBeija getting up on a chair and claiming space as a young Black woman living with HIV. It was toward the end of the event. It was a meta-moment. Here were a bunch of people, mostly white, but not only, in a room debating uses of history when it comes to HIV. Kia expressed that for many of the people in the room the conversation was around meaning and understanding. But for her, it was about her life. She was not the only person living with HIV in the room, obviously, and so what she did for herself and others was to name the fact that AIDS is not an *idea*, it is a condition for people, and in their humanity they need and deserve to be seen, witnessed.

ALEX: That seems exciting and productive.

TED: It was, but I must admit, I have wondered since what could have been different about the event so that a result would have been more people standing up to be seen, or no one having to stand up because everyone felt seen. We were wrestling with real ideas that day: the lure of the past and the lens of nostalgia. Later, it made me think of the David Lowenthal quote that Lucas Hilderbrand uses in his essay "Retroactivism": "What pleases the nostalgist is not just the relic but his own recognition of it, not so much the past itself as its supposed aspirations, less the memory of what actually was than of what was once thought possible."[8]

ALEX: But Ted, back up a second, was Kia's intervention about nostalgia? It seems to me that it was about the present, and how the past was being marshalled (and for whom) in that moment. I know the argument that nostalgia can drain the energy out of the present, but I think there's another use as well, as a way to access insight into the present, calling forth goals or dreams for a better future.

TED: I agree, I do think that Kia's intervention was about the present. I think it was a rebel yell about not falling into nostalgia when consuming media, and the implications that such a fall can take, when much of what was getting remembered at that time failed Black people, and people of color, and women, and so many other people. At a cost to herself, Kia provided us a moment where we were invited to hold then and now together.

ALEX: Ted, is that fair? Are you just protective of Ian and Vincent's work, and maybe thinking through how your event could have better served Kia?

TED: I am. This is why the Revisitation is so exciting and so different than the Second Silence. Like we have said, from 1996 to 2008 things happened, things got made, but the discourse about all this was limited or not at all. This is not the case within the Revisitation. From conversations about erasure to issues around nostalgia, work coming out of the Revisitation is greeted with robust opinions. So much so that I think we can argue that the Revisitation is not the cultural objects alone. Rather, AIDS cultural objects in conversation are the Revisitation.

ALEX: So the Revisitation is not just the (re)turn to AIDS in culture, but the conversation and reactions the work engenders.

TED: Yes, and in fact I think we can argue that as much as it might be an epoch we can mark in time, it is also a process that is now a critical part of the AIDS cultural production and reception.

11 SILENCE + CONVERSATION

1 **SILENCE + YOU**
Think of a time when sharing a struggle, loss, problem, or secret about HIV/AIDS helped you reckon with it. Record or otherwise represent your thoughts.

2 **SILENCE + OTHERS**
Ask someone about a time that they dealt with struggle, loss, a problem, or a secret. Can they represent this? Together, share your stories and/or objects and then discuss the experience of sharing them.

3 **SILENCE + THE WORLD**
Here are three examples of people engaged in conversation and representation arounds AIDS, memory, and vulnerability:
- Group Material. *Democracy: A Project by Group Material*. New York: New Press, 1998.
- Ishmael Houston-Jones, Will Rawls, and Jaime Shearn Coan, eds. *Lost and Found: Dance, New York, HIV/AIDS, Then and Now*. New York: Danspace Project, 2017.
- Nelson Santos, Barbara Schroder, Karen Kelly, and Alex Fialho, eds. *Kia LaBeija and Julie Tolentino in Conversation*. New York: VISUAL AIDS, 2019.

12 SILENCE + INTERACTION

TED: The AIDS Crisis Revisitation is a call and response. It is not only about past citations but also contemporary commentary and plans for the future. It is the fusion of something being done with something being witnessed, and then what happens when all of those forces come together. It is, as we explored in the last chapter, not just the introduction of objects into the culture but the discourse that follows. As we know, many valuable objects were actually produced and introduced within the Second Silence, but they were rarely taken up in culture as had been true during AIDS Crisis Culture, or is true now, within the Revisitation.

ALEX: The Revisitation is not happening within a vacuum. It is unfolding and finding new expression within today's activist communities rooted in feminism, social justice, and equality; in a time deeply informed by anti-Black racism via the Black Lives Matter movement, and the impacts of settler colonialism through the activism at Standing Rock and related #idlenomore activism; the de-silencing around trans experience though unprecedented cultural production; and the inspiring disruptions of the #metoo movement in how we understand gender and power.

TED: Of course, it must be said that all of these forces were in place before the 2016 election of Donald Trump, but in some ways were made more visible and also found kinship in the larger calls to resist: fascism, climate change, or inequality more generally.

ALEX: AIDS is everywhere and sometimes nowhere within these movements, but these movements are ever-present within the Revisitation, either by name or legacy. This is a time when more conversation abounds, due to these and other movements, and both the technologies and despots that have fueled them.

TED: True. We see this in every attempt to remember the past that is deemed too narrowly focused by one audience. But creation occurs in all moments of pushback, each a site of and impetus for new work within the Revisitation.

ALEX: The pushback within the Revisitation, to date, has been largely about race, gender, and in an interesting way, sexuality. The most well-supported and most-discussed works of the Revisitation have been efforts that return to and aim to make sense of AIDS as a twentieth-century plague that was suffered and righted by white gay men. Some of this work suggests that AIDS interrupted earlier gains within the gay rights movement that were then overcome through activism. These works are captivating and inspiring stories of devastating losses and profound wins.

TED: They have been very impactful for me. As a gay white man, I see how we have been and continue to be decimated bodily, emotionally, sexually, and communally by AIDS, and how we have used our access to capital and cultural capital to help ourselves and others through making and supporting work about the past and our relationship to the crisis. That is much of what my early work tried to accomplish. And I am not alone. There are countless examples within the Revisitation of work done by young and youngish gay men dealing with their inheritance of HIV.

ALEX: My work as well. *Video Remains*, while not only or even primarily about a white gay man, is haunted by Jim.

TED: Haunting is a good word, and I think if we look at much of the early Revisitation work, it is artists, filmmakers, curators, and writers doing what you had also done, which is to say, making their mourning productive through cultural production.

ALEX: These films and exhibitions were as much about reaching out to the living as they were about honoring their beloved dead, and the loss of their once tight-knit community of lovers, friends, coconspirators, and witnesses. This work was about healing, for ourselves and our communities.

184

TED: I remember sitting in movie theaters in 2012, the year many of the first major AIDS Crisis Revisitation films were released, and witnessing the anguish of so many people in our community: older, mainly white, mainly male, but not only. At the screening of *United in Anger* at the MoMA, people called out the names of loved ones long dead as they appeared on-screen. Howling and gasps followed. At the Village East Cinema on 12th Street, I had to hold on to the sides of my seat because the shaking and crying during *We Were Here* were so intense. The grief of the thirty or so men gathered in that theater was moving the room's foundation.

ALEX: I saw that film in Los Angeles at Outfest. Not only was it moving to me to be in the large screening room at the DGA when it premiered (the AIDS work that had been screened in previous years was always in the small theater), but the shared mourning was unforgettably cathartic and redemptive.

TED: This was a time of very tender productivity and reckoning. I was working at Visual AIDS and I was part of meaningful and generative cross-cultural and multigenerational conversations, meetings, and events about HIV initiated between the old and the young, and attended by both, and everyone in between. These were totally new. It was also around this time that long-term survivors began to reunite and organize. Some coming out of isolation and others greeting visitors at the proverbial clubhouse door wondering what took everyone else so long to get there. For many people this has been exemplified by the honest, funny, and often heartbreaking writing of Mark King on his influential blog, My Fabulous Disease, where he documents his and other people's experience of living long-term with HIV.[1] Similarly, Lillibeth Gonzalez works with many organizations, including GMHC, to establish public and private forums where people can discuss what it is to be over fifty and both surviving and thriving with HIV.

ALEX: A feeling of waiting to convene was so palpable at the time. There was a sense that much of the audience for these films, and even the makers themselves in some cases, had had some time away from the collective experience of the crisis. And so it is at the end of that interim, and the coalescing of all those private Second Silences, inspired by the gay community's need to heal, that the Revisitation is truly jumpstarted into visibility for large numbers of people. These forces of return, healing, meeting, remembering are then coupled with some communities' real access to resources, as well as individual's personal drive: enough to locate, assemble, distribute, contemplate, and make AIDS history and art (again).

185

TED: Right, and here is where tension enters. The problem was never the circulation of these heartbreaking, informative, beautiful stories of white gay men that were in danger of being lost to history. Rather, the issue was that Western culture is too often driven by the power of one narrative on any given topic. When it comes to HIV, the most visible stories of the epidemic had become (again) about the plight of the gay man, often white, sometimes not.

ALEX: The tension around the space that women, Black people, people of color, trans people and others can take up within the narrative has always been an issue. But as we've established, much of what had been our earliest moves toward diverse representation and inclusion went lost. In the Second Silence, the threads of intersectionality, diversity, and inclusion as tactics to combat the damage of HIV were maintained and passed on, but only in intimate ways.

TED: You are right, and that is a great way of saying it.

ALEX: I know! And I am not even done (although like much of the writing in this book, it was you who wrote that amazing paragraph above!). But I would add, the tactics of survival that are evident in examples like the Bebashi tape did not disappear, they were just held on to, applied, and continued to be marshalled by people who were not in a position of need or want or capacity to look back (yet). In part, this was because the crisis never ended for them, or they had never experienced sustained visibility in the first place. So the idea of a Revisitation never made sense.

TED: So true. This is something Dion Kagan writes about in his 2018 book *Positive Images: Gay Men and HIV/AIDS in the Culture of "Post Crisis,"* in which he thinks about the Revisitation and sees it primarily as a gay white phenomenon, a function of placing the terror of twentieth-century AIDS in the past for communities of gay men who need to move on.[2]

ALEX: Everyone deserves their stories, their memories, their healing, their anger. The issue has been that the preponderance of HIV stories being told about gay white men erases, or at least allows very little air space for, the multitudes of communities impacted by AIDS.

TED: And that is a hard thing to say in public. It can sound as if we are attacking the legitimacy of those stories, or even these men.

ALEX: We are the last people to suggest that anyone can dictate whose story of suffering is worth airing and whose isn't.

TED: But importantly, the overnarrativization of gay men and AIDS doesn't serve us white gay men very well. Overrepresentation leads to pathology. As

Adam Geary points out, a conflation between the gay community and AIDS is rooted in a form of homophobia that ensures that the gay male subject is maintained as a sick identity while perpetuating anti-Black racism.[3]

ALEX: There are lots of ways to be sick, just as there are many ways to be in silence, as well as to remember, record, and share. What we can't deny or forget is that the actual dominant US experience of HIV has been shaped by a hornet's nest of race, sexuality, gender, and linked assertions around who counts as the public in public health. And this divide has always and continues to create disparities along racial, gender, and sexuality lines (and others), with white gay men on one side, and everyone else on the other.

TED: And this is complicated. Age, disability, and class are factors we should consider. *Desert Migration* (Daniel Cardone, 2015) speaks to many of the interlocked issues of aging with HIV, specifically among white gay men.

ALEX: Right, and as you hint at, not only white men. But I want to say that even in whiteness there are material issues of difference being explored in this film. Class and economic status are raised by the film's gay male subjects through its impact on their physical and mental health as long-term, aging survivors. Money is everything when it comes to isolation and access. Some of these men are poor and others wealthy. Their discrete long-term AIDS looks very different in relation to class.

TED: True. I don't think either of us are saying that films about white gay men should be written off. And in fact, I think *Desert Migrations* shows that when we talk about AIDS we are always talking about other issues. The AIDS Crisis Revisitation, for better or worse, highlights and foregrounds how the relationship between difference and dismissal has been part of the crisis all along.

ALEX: Or Ted, as we suggest in Part One, are the definition of the crisis.

TED: True. During the First Silence, a great deal was made of the first five cases of gay men who were reported sick in the *MMRW*, who we only learned later were white. However, very little is made of the next two patients, both of whom were Black, one of whom was not gay. Similarly, we also know that for at least a decade prior to the *MMRW* report, people were dying of "mysterious illnesses" but no reports were filed (that have surfaced), and no alarm set off, as they would be in 1981. In my own work, I research the life of Robert Rayford, a sixteen-year-old Black teenager who died in 1969 with HIV in St. Louis, a fact we know because his saved tissue was tested in 1987 with results

187

published in the *Journal of the American Medical Association* and in mainstream papers the same month. *And The Band Played On* released the myth of Patient Zero to the world.[4]

ALEX: And that myth was coupled with other distortions, themselves fueled by racism, homophobia, and poverty. And it makes sense that while Robert's story has been available to us since 1987, that doesn't always mean that we have been ready or able to deal with it. Revisitation maybe is also an act of mercy, a place of generosity and generative cocreation. It asks us what does it mean to come after? What role do any of us play in being a marshal of the past?

TED: But isn't that exactly what you find frustrating, this act of having to remind people what you and others worked so hard to understand before us?

ALEX: Yes, it is frustrating. But it is also needed. It is the responsible thing to do. And I would be less frustrated by the lift of remembering if I thought it was a more collective pursuit. One of the things I learned coming out of the Second Silence is that we all have a responsibility to tell our stories of AIDS-related experiences—whether these happened in 1981 or 2010. And so I take seriously the job of thinking with work about AIDS, even if there are ethical concerns around it. Take for example *How to Survive A Plague* (2012), by David France, that tracks the lifesaving contributions of ACT UP. By focusing on HIV treatment and related data, they successfully pressured the government to improve access to much-needed medication. This is not an easy film for me to watch. I recognize most of the footage. I had seen it presented when it was made by the people who shot it, my fellow AIDS video activists. I recall seeing it without swelling music or on a large screen. Seeing it now is also hard because I am witnessing dead friends and comrades, and maybe harder still, I am looking for my dead friends and not seeing them. This is devastating. But I know the movie plays an important part in our culture. I know that as much as every frame of that film is already in my bones, it has become something new, and surprising, and upsetting, and empowering for everyone who sees it for the first time. And I hold that along with so much else. I watch for the friends I have lost, but also, I watch it with the friends I have now.

TED: *Like me!*

ALEX: *Like us!* Part of a conversational process is that when I engage in AIDS culture, I am watching with more than one set of senses, with more than one period in mind. I am sometimes consuming with Jim, sometimes with you,

188

sometimes with Juanita, and sometimes with my current batch of AIDS curious students. This is important to me. I am watching this way so that I can be in the dialogue that I longed for within the Silence, as I know you did as well.

TED: I think this is called social viewing, and I do this too! Do you remember that early review I shared with you of *How to Survive a Plague*? The one that I was excited to share with you? It was written on Tumblr, I think, by performance artist Chris Tyler. I asked him about it later, and he explained to me that *How to Survive* reminded him of twenty-first-century superhero movies, like *X-Men* and *The Avengers*: cinematic escape films in which a scrappy but mighty group of underdogs band together to save the world.[5]

ALEX: Yes! And what Chris says rings true. We see it in its most legible form in *How to Survive's* third-act reveal. After we have come to know a world of activists through muddied video footage shot by my friends, our eyes feast upon crisp visions of surviving, male, and predominantly white AIDS activists in the present. These men are my contemporaries. These men are the boys I was a young with. They did great things. But it is hard to see them isolated on the screen. I want to see them with their friends, being hugged, and loved, and in conversation. I can feel the heat of what must have been an intense light on them, and I just want to turn it off.

TED: I dislike those interviews as well, but maybe for less invested reasons. France has discussed how he manipulated the preexisting footage to match those well-lit shots of your friends and comrades.

ALEX: Listen, I am not overly invested in that kind of conversation. Auteurship has never been my thing. I am more interested in what a film does. And let's just say, in its own way, *How to Survive a Plague* is a trigger tape for me, and I mean trigger in the new-school way! Our friend, peer, and fellow AIDS scholar Jih-Fei Cheng is right on in his criticism of the film, always clear to not implicate the survivors, when he writes that *How to Survive a Plague* fetishizes "biological longevity as the end goal to all politics."[6] I love what Jih-Fei does here. A counterintuitive critique of a film about activism maybe, until one remembers that for many, activism is engaged with an awareness that activists themselves may not reap the benefits for which they struggle. For some, especially when activists are from communities not accustomed to state care, those who come after will not easily survive after speaking truth to power.

189

TED: Jih-Fei considers the powerful motivations for those AIDS activists for whom a good life was never guaranteed.

ALEX: That is a useful way of looking at it, and it begins to help build out how the lives of some people with AIDS are intensely different from others.

TED: Which, if we can stay with this a minute longer, is something we should note that Cheng's comments are themselves a part of: his larger project concerning AIDS activist video, specifically around the use of footage. If France's film is focused on the burdens of survival, Cheng is concerned with the afterlife of the AIDS activist dead. Not included in the survivor reveal at the end of the film are Bob Rafsky and Ray Navarro, two enduring presences of the movement who died long before *How to Survive* was made. But as Cheng illustrates, even in passing, equality can be illusive. Yes, as many of us noticed, we get to know Rafsky as a father, gay man, and activist. As we witness him, we see him get sick. His mortality unfolds over time, and as an audience, we are given space to grieve him. In contrast, as Cheng points out, we see Navarro as Jesus twice, and then in a wheelchair. But, unlike with Rafsky, Navarro's illness does not unfold. Navarro gets no eulogy, and we get no time to sit with his passing. We are not even provided the information that Navarro chose to end his life with his mother by his side.

ALEX: The discrepancy in how their deaths are represented is a large part of the film's structural and ethical problem. The way Ray's death plays out in my own *Video Remains* sits in stark opposition. His dear friend and fellow AIDS video activist, Ellen Spiro, narrates to me with pathos, dignity, and honesty about being with him at his bedside as he was dying. In *How to Survive*, Black people, people of color, and people from First Nations are barely seen—and heard from, even less. White women fare a bit better; and trans people are basically not represented at all. When asked about this, France cites a lack of footage.

TED: This is utterly refutable. He got content from activist and videomaker James Wentzy.

ALEX: And all the rest of us.

TED: A quick search of Wentzy's Vimeo page provides a bounty of videos featuring nonwhite people, such as a current favorite among my students: *Native Americans, Two Spirits & HIV* (Wentzy, 1991). This is confusing or troubling. France has spoken about how his goal for the film was to show the lives of the individuals involved in AIDS activism.

190

ALEX: You are being too kind. It is not confusing. But again, I am less invested in what France does, and more interested in the call and response of the film and its viewers within the Revisitation and what comes next when we realize his fundamental blind spots.

TED: Okay, so let's provide a stunning example of this very call and response: the die-in performed by the Tacoma Action Collective (TAC) in response to what they saw as the lack of Black representation in another iteration of the Revisitation, the touring art exhibition, Art AIDS America.

ALEX: Toward the end of the show's first run at the Tacoma Art Museum an inspiring set of demands was released by TAC. Among them is the greater inclusion of Black artists and Black representation as the show moves forward.

ALEX: They demand: "more Black staff at all levels of leadership" at the museum; "Undoing Institutional Racism" retraining for staff and board; and greater Black representation within the Art AIDS America exhibition for when it tours nationally in 2016.[7]

TED: I spoke with curators at various museums along the rest of the Art AIDS America tour. They mentioned how grateful they were for the opportunity to add to the show, in response to the demands that TAC had made. Curators charged with taking the show into their museums across the nation were excited about Art AIDS America and pleased to be given the chance to add local talent.

ALEX: The show had its finale in Chicago at Alphawood, a then brand-new art space. By then, the show was so different from how it began that its curators released a new catalogue.

TED: As part of the Chicago install, a related AIDS exhibition ran at the nearby DuPaul Museum of art. Titled *One Day This Kid Will Get Larger*, the show was curated by Danny Ordenoff and focused primarily on artists born after 1975, with the majority of artists being Black and Brown. (Full disclosure, I had work in the exhibition.)

ALEX: So it is interesting to think about how, as much as you and I might be modeling conversation and responsible Revisitation practices through this book and our individual practices, we can also see TAC as doing the same work in another medium and forum.

191

TED: How do you figure?

ALEX: We'll need to go back a little in time before I get there, if that's okay. Actually, I had never thought about who was in control of managing things from the past as in the same orbit as my feminist AIDS cultural production in the present. But then . . .

TED: I went to Berlin and came back a changed man!

ALEX: If I had a dollar for every time one of my queer friends said that!

TED: Alex! Haha! My Berlin experience was in fact with another man, and as it happens, we were in a basement, sweaty, and my heart was beating. But I must admit, my pants were on, and I was moved less by what he was doing with his body, and more by what was coming out of his mouth!

ALEX: Good one. Go on.

TED: I had just been given a tour of the Schwules Museum in Berlin. A long-time volunteer explained to me the evolution of their collection. It started when archivists were acquiring with the gay experience in mind. It evolved to consider lesbians, bisexuals, and eventually the trans experience. But from the beginning of the known AIDS crisis, the museum collected everything on the subject regardless of identity markers, and as a result, they have an impressive, inclusive, and cohesive HIV archive. It was clear, in his telling, that the museum's trajectory was an emblem of pride. Not only was he proud to be a volunteer with the Museum, he specifically wanted to impress upon me the deep and vast AIDS-related holdings they had. In talking about this, a word came up: stewardship. The museum, he was suggesting, was acting as a steward of an expansive and complex AIDS history, one that early on recognized that the crisis impacted all kinds of folks even amid an implicit collective understanding that AIDS was a gay concern.

ALEX: You were impressed with this idea that underlying a burden of the archive, as he was laying it out, was a notion of responsibility: to represent AIDS not just as it impacted gay, lesbian, bisexual and trans folks, but everyone. To find, save, hold, and share artifacts of all of AIDS history and culture.

TED: Yes, but that it was also okay to start from a place of specificity. As a gay museum, they started collecting AIDS as a form of self-interest, but as the story became more complex they did this work for others, for everyone. It is a reminder that the universal can be in the specific, and that by caring for the specific, you can end up caring for everyone. I was moved by this idea of responsibility that a gay museum understood it had for the public more broadly. Regardless of how widespread AIDS is, and no matter how many communities it impacts, right now a lot of what gets understood as belonging to an AIDS archive exists within LGBTQ frameworks.

ALEX: We will need some really big cultural shifts in where we store and locate AIDS history.

TED: In Norway, for example, Norge-HIV recently donated all their papers to the nation's LQBTQ archive in Bergen. And closer to home, even your own records at the New York Public Library's large holdings of HIV-related papers and artifacts are part of their Gay and Lesbian Collections. Similarly, Story-Corps, which arguably began when the founder interviewed his straight neighbors living with HIV on the Lower East Side about their lives, has an initiative to collect stories about HIV, but this too lives under their LGBTQ initiative.[8]

ALEX: What kind of work can archivists do if their AIDS material resides largely within LGBTQ collections, which is primarily the case?

TED: Archives have a responsibility to liberate information from the often narrow focus of LGBTQ collections. As we have discussed, HIV is as much about race, poverty, gender, and even geography as it is about sexuality and identity. If I had to sum it up, I would say that archives are wise to name the limits of their current classification methods, and then work with independent scholars, donors, academics, and others to cross-reference their holdings as much as possible. I say all this with the experience of knowing many librarians and archivists and seeing first-hand how creative and adaptable they are within their work.

ALEX: So would you say that the kind of AIDS cultural and archival attention we want to understand and even model requires taking collective responsibility? And you see TAC doing that through what we might understand as an intersectional, Black-affirming, relationship to the saving, showing, and honoring of things from the past?

TED: Ha. Yes, but why do I feel like I am being set up for something?

ALEX: Because you are! What you are suggesting archivists and librarians do is something that I am suggesting we can see in TAC's actions!

TED: Taking collective responsibility?

ALEX: Yes! I see them honoring their feelings and knowledge, based on who they are as people living within Black, queer, and intersectional communities, and from their protesting the show out of hope. At a screening of the short film that TAC made about their die-in, Jaleesa Trapp was asked a question about whiteness. She answered by talking about how their work did not come out of a hate for other people, it came out of a love for Black people.

TED: Ah! So the volunteer at the Schwules Museum was able to see how their work was rooted in the gay experience, and then opened up from there. You are suggesting we can see the specificity of TAC's Black love as a powerful and helpful source of what we want from a caring, changing, and ongoing attention to the artifacts of the many Times of AIDS?

ALEX: Yes, and it is not just about the starting point. It is also about the work. If you think about it, TAC could have just written off the *Art AIDS America* exhibition. Or they could have trashed it. We know that it is not the first exhibition in the history of art to fail to meaningfully include Black people, nor the first exhibition in the history of AIDS to do the same. And yet this group of caring and politized people, though their die-in and writing and videomaking, engaged the museum and all the curators involved in the touring exhibition into conversation, with the result being a new approach to remembering and sharing cultural experiences of AIDS that had been failing them but was now, through their care, to be improved for others. TAC cared enough about themselves, their community, the cultural history and ongoing impacts of AIDS, and maybe even the show or parts of the show itself, to not be silent and to do and then also demand better.

TED: When you put it that way, TAC's work becomes that much more amazing. Care is a tactic for social change, but also an organizing and archiving principle.

ALEX: Yes. And we see that in play with Stephen Vider's exhibition *AIDS at Home*, which was up at the Museum of the City of New York.

TED: Vider, as part of his scholarly and curatorial research, is interested in queer domestic relationships, and for him the caring and intimacy that came out of the AIDS crisis has been inspiring and generative.[9] This exhibition explored the many ways that AIDS motivated and constructed ideas around care, such as the creation of the Buddy Program at GMHC, but also informal networks, such as the two gay men who adopted a baby with HIV who were represented in the exhibition via Juanita Mohammed Szczepanski's 1992 video for the Living with AIDS Show, *Two Men and a Baby*. And maybe just as important, *AIDS at Home* was in its own way also another response to the narrow ways HIV was being explored within the Revisitation. Much of the work

194

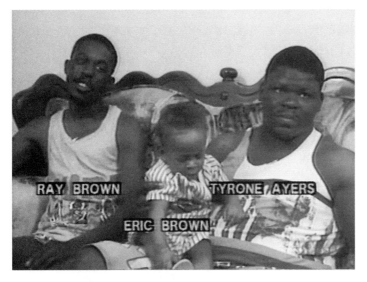

12.1 Frame grab from Juanita Mohammed's Szczepanski's *Two Men and a Baby*, from Caring Sequences (1990, for GMHC's Living with AIDS Show).

was focusing on activism or medicine. To his credit, Vider was interested in returning to the tactic of care as another way of seeing HIV through time.

ALEX: It was an appreciated exhibition, one in conversation with a sister show that I had curated with Hugh Ryan and Jean Carlomusto only months earlier: Everyday in January 2017.[10] I hope it is clear, and we've been reiterating throughout, that ours is a small community of people who work with, learn from, and change discourse together. What was so cool about working with Jean on this show, as well as the videotape we co-curated with Hugh, *Compulsive Practice*, was that this was the first time Jean and I had engaged, not to mention collaborated together, since the tapes we had made together at GMHC in the 1980s. Working with her again was nothing like a repeat. Just as working with you over seven years is not simply more of the same. AIDS had changed, Jean and I were twenty or more years older. The process, output, and focus was new even as Jean and I had always put women, lesbians, and women of color first in our work, given that this was and is the epicenter of trouble for women in the crisis.

TED: Taking time is part of these processes. We know from our own timelines, and our many enduring and inspiring experiences, that change is possible, shifts happen. And that we can be part of these shifts, part of modeling what a real intergenerational relationship to the care of objects, ideas, tactics, and people can be.

195

12 SILENCE + INTERACTION

1 SILENCE + YOU

Locate something you have kept in your possession for a long time. How have you been able to keep it?

2 SILENCE + OTHERS

Bring your object to an encounter with another. Ask them to come with something in hand. What do you need so that you can share your precious things as they deserve?

3 SILENCE + THE WORLD

Here are three works about AIDS and archival practice:

- Marika Cifor. "Your Nostalgia Is Killing Me: Activism, Affect and the Archives of HIV/AIDS." PhD diss., UCLA, 2017. https://escholarship.org/uc/item/2312c9bb.
- Robb Hernández. *Archiving an Epidemic: Art, AIDS, and the Queer Chican/x Avant-Garde*. New York: NYU Press, 2019.
- Cait McKinney. *Information Activism*. Durham, NC: Duke University Press, 2020.

13 SILENCE + TRANSFORMATION

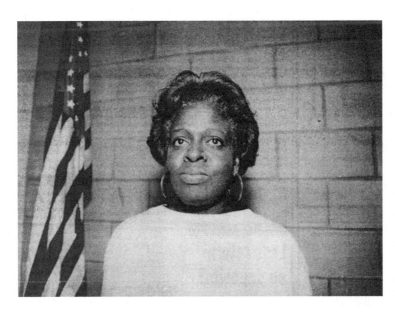

13.1 Joann Walker, from *Metanoia: Transformation through AIDS Archives and Activism,* 2019.

TED: If you walked up to the third floor of the LGBT Community Center of New York City anytime between March 11 and April 29, 2019, you would have been met with a captivating image of an impressive woman.

ALEX: Eyes bright, strong face, her name is Joann Walker, an activist who fought for freedom and humanity for women living with HIV from inside Chowchilla jail in California in the 1990s. An enlarged photograph of her face was the starting point for *Metanoia: Transformation through AIDS Archives and Activism*, an exhibition that we co-curated with educator and filmmaker Katherine Cheairs and organizer and writer Jawanza Williams. Our archival show made use of archival materials that we found at the ONE National Gay & Lesbian Archives at the USC Libraries in Los Angeles and the Center Archive at the LGBT Community Center of New York City.

TED: You were invited by the ONE in Winter 2017 to curate a New York City–based AIDS exhibition building on the success of their Los Angeles exhibition a year earlier, *Lost and Found: Safer Sex Activism*, curated by David Franz and Hannah Grossman. But as is your ethic, one that you were naming and refining with me in the process of writing this book, and one that was responding to the conversation, debates, and drama of the Revisitation, you let it be known that you needed to collaborate on this show. As a white cis HIV-negative woman, even with an extensive history in the movement, and many ideas about AIDS culture, archives, and history that you could certainly draw from, you wanted to collaborate.

ALEX: Although I was worried I might not get the gig, Caitlin McCarthy, the archivist at the Center in New York City, and Jennifer Gregg, who commissioned the show from the ONE, were beyond thrilled when, after informing them not only need I do the show with others, but I could only do a show about stories that still needed to be told from the archive: those of women and people of color. I explained to them that this has always been my core commitment, what I could best contribute, and what was needed in our AIDS activist communities in New York at this time, given the intensity of the critiques of, conversations about, and perceived gaps in the Revisitation.

TED: You brought in three colleagues (including me) from the loose collective in which you and I had also been working on AIDS culture in New York: What Would an HIV/AIDS Doula Do?[1] The four of us knew that to do an exhibition at the Center was an invitation to have influence on the ongoing but transforming Revisitation conversation in our community. To make an argument, our argument.

ALEX: And to engage in processes of curation, exhibition, and remembering; our processes.

TED: To locate and advance ideas and images that would align with the theories that you and I were developing alongside our collective's thoughts about care and community.

198

ALEX: Remember, at this point in our collaboration—yours and mine, Ted— we had done quite a bit of writing, a few public presentations, the two of us together and also with the Doulas, but we had never *made* anything together, we hadn't put these theories about care, archival practices, things, and inter-sectional feminist analysis into practice except as conversation.

TED: At our first gathering, the four of us—who also had never made anything together outside of a successful film screening and public conversation[2]— decided, without any drama or uncertainty, that we were going to center our archival search and show on the activism of Black women living with HIV. We had enough social justice, queer feminism, AIDS, and civil rights knowl-edge between us to understand that by researching in the two host archives around prison and justice, as well as the struggle to change the definition of AIDS, we would find evidence of Black women's experiences and activ-ism even within archives that were not as developed in these areas as any of us might wish. We knew the contributions of Black women could be better shared, witnessed, and circulated through records of their work in both of these activist strongholds, even as both of these archives have not yet had the chance to collect broadly in women of color and HIV.

ALEX: To their credit, Caitlin and Jennifer, who were both commissioning our show, were as aware as were we (if not more so), about legacies within their organizations that had led to patterns of collection and salvage that had, until recently, primarily centered gay white men as the locus of the AIDS story. They were eager to work with us to understand and improve this, find what had actually been saved in their collections, as well as to help us to get to other collections, as needed, and to support us to make new things if and when their archives were not as fertile as we needed to fully center the stories of Black women's response to AIDS.

TED: Don't overlook that at our first meeting we were introduced to what would become perhaps our most important framework.

ALEX: How could I? We were all sharing our backgrounds with each other in AIDS and related movements. We didn't really know each other.

TED: Jawanza showed us the tattoo on his arm, the word "Metanoia" with a cross.

ALEX: Jawanza is a Christian, and Kat and I are not. You are a graduate of seminary with a complex relation to AIDS and spirituality. When he showed us the tattoo, Jawanza told us that AIDS was a transformative agent that had allowed him to become the activist, leader, and man that he is today.

199

TED: This rang true for us as it is at the core of What Would an HIV Doula Do?, the collective that we started in 2015. One of the questions I posed at a one-day gathering ended up becoming our name, What Would an HIV Doula Do? Prior to the symposium, I had been hearing a lot about the work of doulas beyond birth, in terms of end of life, abortion, and gender work. And I was curious about what a doula within the world of HIV could look like. At first it was a very practical idea. But as we began meeting on a monthly basis and continued to talk, it was clear that a doula is a role that already existed within and around us, and just needed to be named as such and then also valued. Through that work we came up with a definition of who we were and what we hoped to do: a doula is someone who holds space during times of transition and HIV is a series of transitions that begin long before any test, and long after treatment.

ALEX: Which is what drew me to the group. In my own life I have seen HIV change over time, and I have seen HIV change people and society.

TED: *Metanoia* seemed more than perfect as a framework to name our doula work, activism, archival work, which we hoped to do together.

ALEX: For our exhibition, Jawanza wrote:

> Metanoia is the first word that I've learned that articulates fully the transformative nature of movement work. AIDS required a movement to address the issue, and still does, and the archives substantiate that something as devastating as AIDS, racism, sexism, and imprisonment are catalysts for movements to build a new world.

From Jawanza we also learned that metanoia is a Greek word that means transformation.

TED: Curating this exhibition, the question became, how can an exhibition hold space? How can an exhibition lead to transformation?

ALEX: This seemed easy to answer: you act generously with information. You claim responsibility but not expertise. The past and the present work together. You let others lead when they are asking to or are the most qualified. From there you offer what you know, ask questions, offer information and sources, and keep the process open.

TED: Which is what we did. And in the process, as Kat would say, the work found us.

ALEX: You were not there, but I was at the Center's Archive with Kat when she opened the box from the Judy Greenspan Archive and first came across an image and mention of Joann. For Kat, it was like the archives were talking to her, to us. Thankfully she listened and we knew that it was right to follow Kat's lead. Over time, we learned that the woman whose picture called to Kat was an activist, a Black woman living with HIV who, while incarcerated for the petty crime of stealing a jacket, helped to free women from jail who were dying with HIV, successfully arguing for their (and ultimately her own) compassionate release. Her work from the inside drew the outside's attention to the deplorable conditions that women and all people living with HIV were dealing with in prison. She helped transform people's lives (including her own), the conditions in the jail, and the terms and foci of activism that was taking place.

TED: This practice of letting the archives speak to you is one shared by many people who do this work. But doing this as a group of four diverse people (and under a very tight deadline), was as much about the excitement in what we were finding as it was a kind of awe around the stories we were able to find and then share. It was also a reminder, relying on a sense of solidarity built over time, that intersectional work around HIV has not only been happening since early on, it has also been documented, circulated, celebrated, and so on.

ALEX: I was in the *Center's Archive* when Kat opened a cardboard box and encountered Judy, then met Joann, and was later introduced to Twillah, all women who are central to the story we tell in *Metanoia*. Each time, she responded bodily. I felt it, too, in the room. I heard her vocalize from across the table in the hushed room. It was electric, and deep. Later, she came to where I was seated and explained what had happened. I already knew. The people who are held in the archive were the women Kat needed to know. I was honored and changed by being allowed to witness these introductions.

TED: If we, as a crew, were going to take seriously our roles then we had to listen to what the archive was providing, and think about that content as it related to the stories we felt called to share. Along the way we came across, and got to know, people, tactics, and politics that inspired us. In turn, their work informed our own processes of curating and collaboration and reflected back to us our commitments. Meeting these women was transforming us as individuals and as a collaborative.

ALEX: Any exhibition that any one of us would have done on our own would have been in that political wheelhouse, but collectively as four individuals who also interacted lovingly with the archive and its people as partners, we came up with ideas, findings, frameworks, and connections that were beyond any of our singular capacities, and beyond what you and I alone had been able to do as writing-partners to date.

TED: Collaborating with Kat and Jawanza was part of this, opening our conversations in new directions and consolidating them in others: another cisgender male and female working with us; another gay man and queer woman in the mix; two people who were in slightly different generations from ours; two more AIDS activists with their own educations, histories, commitments; two African Americans; a collaborator who is living with HIV.

ALEX: I'm not going to pretend this was easy! Writing, building conservation, and curation across four people was more than twice as hard as doing it between the two of us. Rough patches, different interpretations, intensity, the pressure and possibility of difference are all productive in the AIDS Response as long as they occur in community and with care.

TED: In the process of the exhibition—you know, you were there—I experienced a break, a set of freak-outs if you will, in which during more than one curatorial meeting I was overcome by emotion and had to leave the room.

ALEX: This was really hard for all of us, because in our community, in our small circles, even between just you and me, you are always our rock: ethical, kind, smart, sensitive.

TED: It was amazing how the three of you held space for me.

ALEX: That wasn't hard. We let you have your intense feelings even as we never fully understood why you were having them.

TED: That was because I wasn't sure what was happening. But with some time, it seems clear that my intense emotional response to our process making this show was a result of much of the conversation that we had in this book.

ALEX: I'm surprised to hear you say that. We might have thought it would have prepared you.

TED: Trauma is always present in AIDS work, just as is pleasure, friendship, and power. As a white gay man, coming of age in the face of AIDS, my own differences from the three of you felt very live to me on those occasions.

ALEX: But that's why we love you, and want to work with you! Your differences make us wiser. Your commitments ground us.

TED: That's more or less what you said in your writing for the exhibition:

> Our difference is one of our gifts, a most gracious and generative thing that we can share. None of us are alike. Not in age, race, sexuality, birthplace, education, HIV status, or spirit. We are surrounded by powerful divisive forces—tyrants, corporations, nations, homophobes, racists, and some of us, prison walls—and yet, we can also strive to be surrounded and abetted by our glorious differences, and connections, through our art, records, conversations, daily living and activism.

I'd like to add another place where our differences were key to understanding changing patterns in the AIDS Response. Of course, our show, like so many others in the past few years, can be seen as a response to earlier curatorial work within the Revisitation. On the most obvious level, our show was not about white gay men living and dying with HIV in LA, New York City, and San Francisco. But harder to say is that it was not rooted in not being about something.

ALEX: Double negative! Do you mean we weren't on the defensive; that we were newly open to being proactive? That enough of that negative or defensive reaction had been done by us, and others, so that we could be liberated to say and show what we believed in, but not as a critique or a correction of someone else's effort? If so, then yes! *Metanoia* was rooted in Black women's power, pleasure, pain, and defiance. It was mounted for other Black women, and for the AIDS community more generally, who had much to learn from this less-well-known perspective on AIDS culture and history.

TED: The show was not in a usual gallery; rather, it was in the halls and on the walls of the LGBT Center in New York City, which has over six thousand visitors a week.

ALEX: It was exciting and an honor and a challenge to reach out to this broad queer community about our very specific slice of the AIDS story.

TED: Most of these people are there attending one of the twelve thousand yearly meetings or events hosted at the center including readings, speed dating, and AA, NA, and other related meetings. Plus there were people using the space because it has heat in the winter, air conditioning in the summer, accessible bathrooms, computers, a coffee shop, and other people to hang out with and see.

ALEX: We kept reaffirming to each other that it was "for the people in the center's hallways" who we made the show: people we knew had some relationship to HIV by virtue of being part of the LGBTQ community in the United States, and people who for the most part might not have seen a lot of AIDS exhibitions. But remember, we also would say, what about the white gay dudes? How are they going to take this?

TED: And then we would say, either they won't engage, or they will take this in, and won't that be part of the good work we are hoping to do! Let's work with them to understand how Black women's experience of HIV will enrich their own. Which is to say, not through a medical, scientific, or even an art or prevention lens, but through the experiences, desires, practices, activism, and analyses of Black women who have much to express and reveal.

ALEX: Which meant among many things that people who we wanted to plug into the show (as workers and contributors in a variety of capacities) who were Black, who were women, did not have to go through translation into their expression. Our show was about and for Black women. It was audiences from outside this community who would need to be open to that kind of translation work, and perhaps the show could help.

TED: Which brings us full circle, doesn't it? As it happened, Part One of this book was written before and during the run of *Metanoia* in New York. For me, our process for creating *Metanoia* became deeply rooted in and informed by watching and writing about the Bebashi tape, in seeing AIDS work from some Black women from the past and thinking about the arguments they were making with their art, the processes they were engendering, and the ideas of audience and interaction that we learned from them.

ALEX: Me too. There is real connective tissue between the women of Bebashi and Joann Walker, well beyond their experiences as Black women dealing with HIV. They are also mediamakers and activists using their voices to help others and themselves.

TED: They were all activists who situated their work primarily in community.

ALEX: Among the most engaging photos of the exhibition was an image of activist Katrina Haslip, who is also a sister to these women.

TED: She is best known for her activism as a person living with HIV, who worked with others to help change the definition of AIDS. It is not until 1993, after years of various approaches—from direct action to lawsuits—that the

204

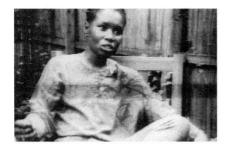

13.2 Frame grab, Katrina Haslip, *I'm You, You're Me: Women Surviving Prison, Living with AIDS,* Catherine Saalfield [Gund] and Debra Levine, 1992.

US government opened up the definition of AIDS to include more of the opportunistic infections that were impacting many people who were not able to be named as living with AIDS—such as cis women—because their infections did not present as the same illnesses that men were suffering from. Outside of its poor science and glaring sexism, this was critical at that time because an AIDS diagnosis was not only a recognition of what someone was going through health-wise, it was also a key to unlocking opportunities, such as eligibility for drug trails and access to resources that would reduce the burden of the illness while the person was still alive as well as for the family after death. Because of the history and science of HIV being primarily understood as a disease impacting gay cis men, much of the knowledge production, including definitions, retained and were made from that bias. To call it out and change it has always been the work of AIDS activists, such as Katrina. She was at the New York State prison, Bedford Hills, where she was a mentor to many, helping to create ACE (AIDS Counseling and Education Program), and training herself to become a jailhouse lawyer. Working with lawyer Terry McGovern on the outside, and members of the National ACT UP Women's Committee and the New York ACT UP CDC Committee, Katrina sued the Office of Social Services calling out the AIDS definition as deficient because it did not include women. It was this case, along with associated demonstrations in Atlanta, Los Angeles, and elsewhere, that led to the AIDS definition being changed in 1993. We told this archival story in our show as well. One of power as well as loss. Katrina did not live long enough to benefit from her own work. She died in late 1992.

ALEX: This is a somber reminder that activism is slow and hard. All of this communal care, duration, attention, and action is documented in the 1992 ACT UP Women's Committee book *Women AIDS and Activism*[3] as well as the more recent 2017 film, *Nothing without Us: The Women Who Will End AIDS,* a film by Harriet Hirshorn. People can learn more about ACE and the work

205

Katrina and other women did about HIV in prison in a video by Catherine Saalfield [Gund] and Debra Levine, *I'm You, You're Me: Women Surviving Prison* (1992). We showed this video with four others about women, prison justice reform, and HIV as part of *Metanoia* programming in New York City.

TED: As these videos attest, Katrina was such a powerhouse, and there is such good footage that documents that about her. I am honestly confused about how and why she does not yet take up more space in the Revisitation. Where is *her* feature film?

ALEX: But is that the goal? I think one of the themes of this book when it comes to media, archives, AIDS, and activism is that bigger might at first seem better, and that more audience views may result in greater recirculation in the future, but that is not always true nor always the best goal. There are different textures and even knowledges that come with media of various sizes, scope, and reach. Sure, it would be great if everyone knew Katrina's name, but to what ends? As it is now, we can see how learning about Katrina, Joann, and Bebashi via interventions like short videos, this book, and our exhibition can lead to a different type of attachment for different communities and with that, the possibilities for a thicker bonds to form between legacies, people, and the present. Does that make sense?

TED: Yes, I see what you are saying, and I am thinking back to a panel that I was on when I asked the audience why people know Larry Kramer's name and not Katrina's. Rhetorically this was a fine gesture, and proved a point about white supremacy and misogyny. But it is not exactly indicative of my work or our work or larger commitments. I am not trying to erase Larry or his work; I just want more diversity in what is known, remembered, and what is possible when it comes to the stories we tell about HIV—past, present, and future.

ALEX: Katrina may one day take up the space in culture that Larry does. We don't know. But fame of this sort is not the marker that matters most to me of success, or value, or change. But also, Ted, let's not forget, our opening was huge! Remember the female drummers, the many speeches, the dancing, the food! We had media attention, and we were invited to move the show to LA.

TED: The opening was wonderful: a physical gathering in which we could see and engage with, all in one place, the various people, communities, and influences that care about and inform the work we do.

206

ALEX: Things on a wall have only so much power. Until they are looked at, paid attention to, and brought into discussion, they are lonely if proud objects. On this, I loved how Kat wrote about the power of objects and archives for our show:

> Archives are living, breathing objects. A letter, flyers, newspaper article, or poster carries the energy, history, and soul fire of the time from which they originated. The archive is a who done it; an unsolved mystery whose story unfolds in your hands. Archives make you laugh. Archives make you cry. Archives soothe the ache of a place you cannot name. Archives reflect the continuum of your life with the others that came before and who will come after.

TED: Yeah, that is lovely. In thinking about that, what is your favorite way we brought the archives to life?

ALEX: Well, I liked the letters the four of us mounted on the wall from Joann to Judy, and I am very proud of our AIDS poster curation that was peppered throughout the exhibition from the Center and One's extensive collections focusing, again, on their holdings about Black women and community. But I think the most generous work we did was the finding and exhibition of the chants. While sharing the contributions of Katrina and Joann is one clear example of recovery, the chants seemed generous in a different way.

TED: I did a lot of tours during the run of the exhibition, and the chants were always the most discussed. On a tour I did for Visual AIDS, Brian Carmicheal, a writer, artist, and activist who had been on the inside for a while, talked about how meaningful hearing the chants had been when he was in jail in the 1990s. They made him feel less alone. He said the same about receiving letters.

ALEX: That is so nice to hear, and something that rings true for me. I love going to a march to put my body on the line, knowing that I am going to be fed and fueled by my community. The physical work of marching is part of that, but for me, so too is unison chanting, and the call and response.

TED: Funny you say that. On another tour, a seasoned activist spoke about how they see chants as the most crucial and successful form of popular education. Complex ideas are simplified into joyous and clear words and demands that can be easily communicated.

ALEX: All of that. So I have to say my favorite part of the opening was how we activated the chants. We asked the crowd to perform together some of the chants we had found in the archive that were written for actions about women in prison. When we chanted these together at our opening, we were

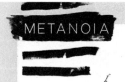

1. WOMEN DIE, THEY DO NOTHING

2. IF YOU'RE POOR OR A WOMAN, ITS NO SURPRISE
   ~~ITS NO SURPRISE~~, CORPORATE MEDICINE IS TELLING YOU LIES

3. AIDS DEFINITION NEEDS CORRECTION,
   ADD TO THE LIST VAGINAL INFECTION

4. HEY, HEY, C.DC.,
   WHEN WILL YOU RESEARCH P.I.D.

5. HEALTH CARE IS A **RIGHT**,
   NOT JUST FOR THE STRAIGHT MALE WHITE

6. JUST SAY NO is what the Bigots preach,
   NO SEX, NO DRUGS + NOT FREE SPEECH

7. C.D.C. YOU FUCKING SCUM,
   WHY DON'T YOU RESEARCH WIMMIN'S CUM

8. LESBIANS HAVE SEX

9. LESBIANS GET AIDS.

10. WIMMIN WITH AIDS CAN'T WAIT TIL LATER
    WE'RE NOT YOUR FUCKING INCUBATORS

13.3 ACT UP/LA chants from the 1990s, distributed by the ACT UP national women's caucus. The chants were found by *Metanoia* curators in the Judy Sisneros / ACT UP LA papers at the ONE Archive.

all focused together, with one voice, on Black women's bodies, women's sexuality, and women in prison. I felt the transformational power of this in a way that I rarely have. As we chanted together, we were one community of sound and body, brought together by AIDS and Black women! A different kind of conversation, right, Ted? There we were, all dressed up, surrounded by many of the people represented and involved in the show, as well as funders, including the older white gay men who had contributed generously to the Center, the ONE, and this show! And to hear them not only say "vaginal infection," but repeat it, was just wonderful. I think it is so critical to name that there has been a way that the Revisitation has played out that has gone on to leave gay white men feeling like their pain, their contributions, their legacies have to be sidelined. That has been hard to witness. What our opening reflected is that their experiences can be seen and honored differently when we let other centers of gravity create new loci for the AIDS Response. Their voices, and histories, can also be heard when they join in our struggle, pain, and infection.

TED: Also, it should be noted, there was no graffiti or wear and tear on any of the work, except for the chants. Someone crossed out the word "FUCK" on one of them.

ALEX: Oh Ted! I love that. Not because of censorship, but rather, yet again the proof of engagement and interaction in the face of Revisitation. Someone was reading, feeling, and reacting. In terms of engagement, what was your favorite?

TED: I loved the lesson plan that educator Lavern McDonald made for her Punishment, Politics, and Culture class for Calhoun High School (for queer youth). She taught about the exhibition by taking in Katrina and Joann's story and then contextualizing it within a lesson plan for her students. To me this means that we were clear enough in our collaborative archival work that someone else was able to pay it forward. I was happy we included it in the guidebook, along with a beautiful essay by archivist Steven G. Fullwood.

ALEX: That is something the four of us did well. We knew that to make the work live we had to share it and include even more people.

TED: And we had to help people connect registers of time. As much as Katrina and Joann's work is in the past, it is with us today in multiple ways, including as something to learn from and see ongoing.

209

ALEX: Which gets us to one of the other exciting parts of the exhibition: the commissioned photographs by Lolita Lens taken of Nathylin Flowers

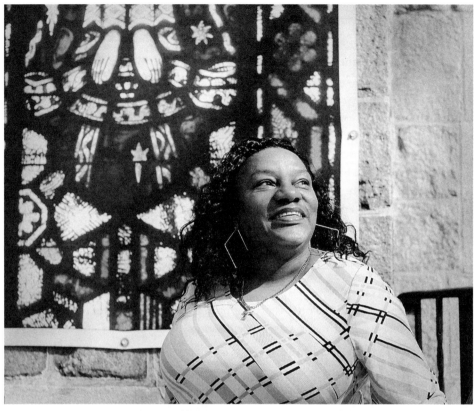
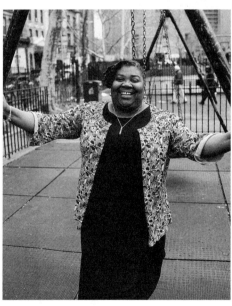
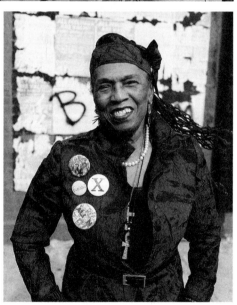

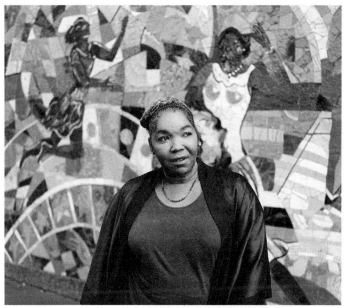

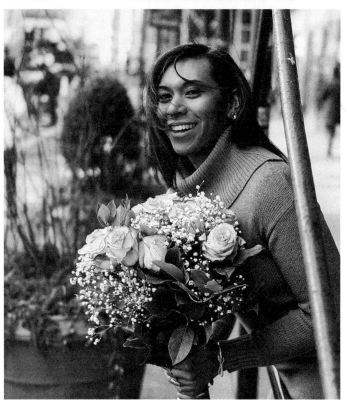

13.4–13.8
Collage of photos of the New York City activists, taken by Lolita Lens. Opposite: Shirlene Cooper (*top*), Rusti Miller-Hill (*bottom, left*), Nathylin Flowers Adesegun (*bottom, right*); Adjacent: Kiara St. James (*top*), Malaya Manacop (*bottom*).

Adesegun, Shirlene Cooper, Malaya Manacop, Rusti Miller-Hill, and Kiara St. James, all Black and women of color activists working today in the intersectional fields of HIV, gender, race, and incarceration. Here's how we manifested, yet again, our fundamental commitment to the present. We linked their work today with archival materials, all on the wall, and then in our tours, we enlivened the past's activists through this connection.

TED: That aspect of the show is beyond beautiful.

ALEX: Again, this was Kat following her intuition. We had named a few photographers we wanted to work with, but had not landed on one who clicked. Kat went online and found Lolita Lens in a Facebook group for Black female photographers.

TED: Together we created a list of women who we knew were doing good work, and then we brought the artist and the activists together!

ALEX: Right, and then when we were being interviewed live on the radio we learned that Rusti knew Katrina and that she had been a powerful influence in her life.

TED: Something you can't really tell from the documentation of the work is that these images were in a long narrow hallway across from message boards: old-school, pre-internet, message boards where people advertise jobs, housing needs, upcoming culture, and the like. I really loved how the community activists were part of this vibe, this idea of old-school outreach and communication.

ALEX: That's why we had to include ourselves and our own process in the show, on the same walls.

TED: I would often start or end the tours with reading my own statement and then having others read all of your statements to give voice, since you were not there. It was a way of acknowledging and honoring everyone's contributions, and thinking about the various ways we can bring voice into the work, even for people not present with us in any given room.

ALEX AND TED: So here's Kat's:

> I followed an intuitive hunch. The Judy Greenspan papers in the
> finding aid at the Center had a few subject headings: Women, Prison,
> California. Thinking there might be the stories of women of color ly-
> ing there, I began searching through the Greenspan archive. My first
> sighting of Joann Walker was on the cover of a Fire Inside Newsletter.

212

Looking closely at her small photo included in the article, Walker's assured gaze pierced straight to my soul. I thought, "Is this the Ida B. Wells of this work in Chowchilla?" A later conversation with Greenspan confirmed this as true. Finding Joann's articles, poems, personal letters, and photos has changed my life. After my visit to the Center, I lay down that night and said, "Thank you, Joann Walker; you are not forgotten; we say your name; we honor you."

TED: This piece of writing from Kat demystifies the archival process and illustrates how so much research is showing up to the tedious work of looking and then availing oneself of what the content offers. I think Kat would be the first to declare that moment in the archive, that you described earlier, as the start of the metanoia magic. There was a way in which the lives of the people we were meeting in the archives was dovetailing with our own experiences.

TED AND ALEX: As we saw with Jawanza's entry as well:

Because of my own experience living with HIV and organizing with a powerbuilding grassroots organization committed to ending AIDS, I knew that exploring the contributions of Black women and femmes in the political response to AIDS would be interesting and critical for a comprehensive, nuanced reclamation of power, and who is remembered for building it. AIDS is the only illness that required a sociopolitical movement that ultimately transformed the United States in measurable and phenomenological ways.

Exploring Joann Walker's story through her archives and uncovering ephemera in the Greenspan archives affirmed many of my thoughts about the power of organizing, AIDS, gender, and the carceral state to produce the conditions that kill people, but also, initiate a psycho-socio political process that is part and parcel to moving the world toward a quality and condition that is more humane and just. I organize daily to recreate the sort of activation we find with Joann's work around women's healthcare in prisons because I believe that these are the things that produce *Metanoia*, the things that push us beyond suffering and into action.

TED: I am curious about how, after all we have said about the AIDS Crisis Revisitation, you think we can fit in our exhibition.

ALEX: Ted! Are we really having this conversation again? Is this the rest of our lives, you asking me how something fits into the Revisitation?

213

TED: On some level, yes, I guess. Ha! But for real, part of our conversations is about asserting that not all AIDS culture is about the past, and that has been hugely important to me. I think it is important to assert that AIDS culture can be about the present, and maybe on some level is always about the present because of reception.

ALEX: The Revisitation holds all the Times of AIDS. It has put AIDS back into time because it brings the past into dialogue with the present: it is texts and also the conversations they generate. Within the ongoing AIDS Crisis Revisitation, people are doing what we did with *Metanoia*, freeing themselves from looking at the same artists, cities, communities, posters, and slogans that have been seen so many times and bringing new voices, histories, people, communities, art, and frameworks into the visible Times of AIDS.

TED: In the process of writing this book, I realize that is my life goal. To help the world divest from narrow collective conversations about AIDS, and to better broaden the discussion to strive toward comprehensiveness: to include everything that has ever been said and open up to everything that has not yet been said once, twice, or heard a million times.

ALEX: Wow. What a life goal, Ted. One foot in the past and the other in the future, with the will to full inclusion and deep diversity in the present, so as to share information and inspiration that was made before and is useful now.

THIRTEEN. SILENCE

13 SILENCE + TRANSFORMATION

1 **SILENCE + YOU**
How has your relationship to or understanding of AIDS been impacted over the course of this book? How have you been transformed? Represent this.

2 **SILENCE + OTHERS**
How or where can you preserve your representation of your transformation? How will you share this?

3 **SILENCE + THE WORLD**
Here are four online AIDS archives:
- African American AIDS Activism Oral History Project. https://web.archive.org/web/20180611031008/https://afamaidsoralhistory.wordpress.com/.
- Gay and Lesbian Collections and AIDS/HIV Collections, New York Public Library. https://www.nypl.org/lgbtqcollections.
- HIV/AIDS Caregivers Oral History Project. https://archives.lib.umn.edu/repositories/13/resources/2123.
- Visual Arts and the AIDS Epidemic: An Oral History Project. https://www.aaa.si.edu/inside-the-archives/visual-arts-and-the-aids-epidemic-oral-history-project.

CONCLUSION

WE ARE BEGINNING THIS CONVERSATION, AGAIN

In the winter of 2020, asynchronously on our laptops, we watched the documentary *Can You Bring It? Bill T. Jones and D-Man in the Waters* (Rosalynde Le-Blanc and Tom Hurwitz, 2020). The film is marketed as "a love story between dancers Bill T. Jones and Arnie Zane, and the diverse dance company they founded." Their love is there, everywhere, but so too is love between their original dance troupe and for these two men. Amid all this feeling is a critical examination of one signature dance, "D-Man in the Water," a stunning and significant work from AIDS Crisis Culture, and an enduring (and we will soon see, changing) testament to artmaking as a way to heal, rage, create community, and consider the ongoing register of AIDS's impact and trauma.

The dance was the first work the company created after cofounder and choreographer, Arnie Zane, died of AIDS within the arms of his community. The film documents a restaging of the piece, thirty years later, by LeBlanc, one of its original dancers, now a professor and choreographer, and also a codirector of the documentary. We watch her revisit a dance she knows from inside out, making it again, newly, with a troupe of her students at Loyola Marymount University in Los Angeles. Their present-day process is cut against documentary footage of the original dance and present-day interviews with Jones and his dancers who remember and testify to its origin, as well as its legacy. The tension at the heart of this otherwise tranquil and kind film is around how and if one can make the trauma of AIDS, the loss of loved ones, relevant enough to today's dancers that the piece can work:

feel inspired, have power, be true to what it once meant and did, and stay true to what it can accomplish in this Time of AIDS. How do you make AIDS work from the past work in the present? In LeBlanc's pursuit to transmit the choreography and context of the dance, she brings in Jones, who carries with him the movements and memories in his body, which embodies the past and present of the dance and of HIV/AIDS for her students.

This documentary serves as a powerful end to our book because in the film we see all our Times of AIDS as well as what we suggest is a new one, the one we are both living in and trying to understand now, as we finish this lengthy project. AIDS Before AIDS is represented with a seemingly off-the-cuff remark by Jones about the timing of his and Zane's arrival in New York City in the late 1970s. Here was a world rich with a robust and teeming gay sexual culture, which was, he admits with hindsight, maybe not so wonderful considering "what was to come." AIDS is there, anticipated, unknown, unseen, yet palpable to us now. The First Silence is represented through a montage of newspaper headlines from the early 1980s documenting the mounting crisis, intercut with a clip of President Reagan heartlessly preaching about morality.

AIDS Crisis Culture takes up the bulk of the film's first half. Through interviews with the surviving members of the troupe—and as powerfully through footage of this time haunted by our understanding that nearly half of them died—we are invited to be with them in the New York dance scene and the intensity and inescapable impact of AIDS in the late 1980s and early 1990s. We see a brief clip of Zane working from home in the last weeks of his life as he continues to make work, to dance and to teach, even as he maneuvers an IV drip on a pole and wheels.

We learn that "D-Man in the Waters" was a collective creation facilitated by Jones in the aftermath of Zane's death. Just as the women of Bebashi came together to make a video about how to live and die within a pandemic, using their own experiences and bodies as a tool for themselves and others in a process they determined, so too did the Bill T. Jones/Arnie Zane Dance Company. Through structured interactions and a building language of choreography, the company mined their lives and losses for movement, expressing the looming presence of illness and death in their bodies and community. But as Jones names in the film, they also danced to express "a joy for survival." As is true for other works made during AIDS Crisis Culture, "D-Man in the Waters" has become canon. It is the troupe's most performed piece to this day. Made to make the AIDS crisis legible in its Time, it stays visible in ours.

The Second Silence is rendered in the film through gaps. The name of the dance, "D-Man," is the nickname given to Demian Acquavella, a young and

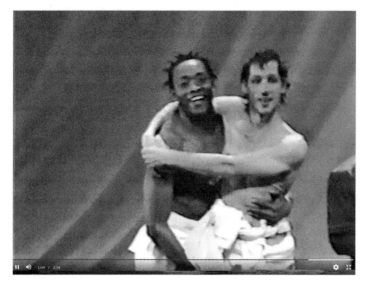

C.1 Jones and Acquavella during the curtain call with Arthur Ailes (still from *Can You Bring It? Bill T. Jones and D-Man in the Waters*, 2020).

new member of the troupe. But by the time the work debuts at the Joyce, we learn that D-Man is living in a body so ravaged by the virus and lack of available treatment that he can't perform. Instead, he participates on stage for one special event. While he lays immobile on the stage, Jones invents ways to dance with him. At the end of the performance, Jones carries Acquavella onto the stage for the curtain call. It is D-Man's last performance before his death.

When LeBlanc chooses to restage this dance, she embarks on a Revisitation project not unlike what Alex did with *Video Remains*. What can be done with historic, perhaps even dated material—be it footage or choreography—that draws forward the past for ongoing uses: memorial, education, conversation, healing, and world-building?

In watching the film alone and together, what struck us both was that as much as it was about and rooted in the past, at some point it stopped being about revisitation, and started being—we think—about what becomes possible beyond simply looking back. What happens after Revisitation?

COMING INTO [CRISIS] NORMALIZATION

In the winter of 2019, together in a theater, we saw *One in Two*, a play by Donja Love. The work is rooted in both his decades-long journey of living with HIV and the CDC statistic that one in two Black gay men will receive a positive diagnosis in their lifetime. With this statistic in mind, the audience

219

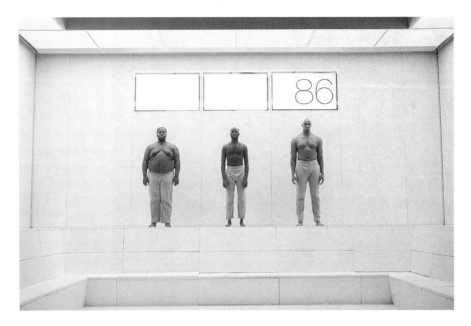

C.2 *One in Two*, by Donja Love.

watches as three Black gay men play at diagnosis, each taking turns as they imagine and understand the implications of "what if?"

We both loved the play. As we discussed it, we wondered where it fit in our Times of AIDS. As we will soon get into—demonstrating our ongoing process of knowing and naming Times—it was, we realized, something new. A new or different Time that we have come to call AIDS [Crisis] Normalization.

The play takes advantage of the fact that in this sixth time of AIDS that we are proposing, the epidemic is established and known, and thus no longer positioned as a collective crisis. Removed from these previously definitive conditions for AIDS cultural production, in *One in Two*, AIDS is afforded space to be considered without having to be a fight for visibility within silence, or as something defined against or via a brutalizing history. While it is clear that the past informs Love's play, *One in Two* is about AIDS in the present. This was another clear sign of something we had already begun to name: over the time we were writing this book, AIDS had gone from something we had to look for in cultural production to an increasingly stable part of everyday experience. We realized that over the last seven years, a mention of AIDS may have even come to be expected, or at least less noteworthy. We had once texted each other any time we stumbled upon a crumb of AIDS in cultural production.

By the time we came to write this conclusion, that was neither possible nor inspiring. There's just too much work for any inclusion of AIDS to matter in and of itself.

One example of this from a few years ago is in the first season of the ABC legal thriller *How to Get Away with Murder*, produced by Shonda Rhimes. Series regular Oliver (Conrad Ricamora) is diagnosed with HIV. As far as disclosure goes, the stigma attached to this diagnosis is in keeping with primetime soaps: just dramatic enough. A year later, PrEP is introduced into the storyline as Oliver begins a relationship with Connor (Jack Falahee), an HIV-negative man. By 2018, Oliver shares with his mother his positive HIV status. During the show's run (which ended in 2020), the most remarkable thing about the HIV storyline was just how unremarkable it was.

In this TV series, HIV is integrated in the show's narrative alongside other aspects of characters' lives. Audience commentary on social media takes on the inclusion of HIV, but it is not the dominant concern. It seems that AIDS is again—or maybe for the first time in history—understood as part of the fabric of the story and the society in which that story is set. The inclusion of the epidemic into other dramatic arcs puts AIDS into a new place: visible but not spectacular; critical but not a [Crisis].

Finding ourselves within a new time of AIDS was exciting and nerve-racking. As part of our process, we began to slowly build a list of outliers as well as a taxonomy of what made these works similar to each other, and different from but connected to work from the previous Times of AIDS. From there, by paying attention to *One in Two*, *How To Get Away with Murder*, *Can You Bring It?*, and other works,[1] we began to name that AIDS [Crisis] Normalization:

- situates HIV as one of many concerns;
- presents HIV stigma, and yet this may be less connected to historic and ongoing homophobia, trans, or queerphobia;
- is present-focused and present-invested (while the past can still be informative);
- may (or may not) include mass death, untreatable illness, and early hallmarks of the epidemic, but either way, is not primarily rooted in trauma.

Notable within AIDS [Crisis] Normalization work is a message that AIDS is not over, even if the urgent, angry, awful inspirations of previous generations begin to recede or even disappear; even if disclosure never happens; 221 even if HIV is undetectable; even if saying "AIDS is over" is also a mantra of this Time. But AIDS remains, as does crisis, even as all this becomes less formative or visible. We attempt to represent this new epoch of visibility in the structure of our term: AIDS [Crisis] Normalization. We include the word "crisis" between square brackets, a symbol that indicates an easily missed, almost forgotten presence: there and not there, effecting what comes before and after it, but doing so gently, quietly, while maintaining a magnetic pull. Our poetic use of punctuation indicates that while AIDS might be stabilizing in important ways within the culture, it remains an acute and daily crisis for many, and an open and unresolved issue for the culture as a whole.

Today, as has been true across all the Times of AIDS, HIV is a highly stigmatized illness that disproportionately burdens communities neglected and hurt by systems that should be designated for care and service. Because of systemic neglect, some people with HIV continue to die. Medicine, policies, and even culture is only as good as it is accessible. This is true, or maybe especially true, within this period we are calling Normalization because the disparity between those who are "AIDS-free" and those for whom it continues as a crisis is ever more intense. While HIV takes up a more consistent and even expected place in culture, it is still a wound, an open question, an experience in need of representation, action, and justice.

Normalization is not inherently good. For many of us, the cultural impact of what is considered normal has been stifling, oppressive, and worse. As we have seen, given that racism is normal, its normalization will be toxic and violent. One of the assumptions of this book is that AIDS Times emerge from silence and are rooted in trauma. Central to AIDS Crisis Culture is mass death and neglect; central to the AIDS Crisis Revisitation is a trauma-informed call to not forget. Normalization is a result of how AIDS communities used the beautiful, intense, voluminous work of all the Times of AIDS, including the Revisitation, to attend to, in a variety of ways and across a range of formats, the traumas of AIDS, including those produced by the First and Second Silence. These traumas—and the losses of life, suffering, grief, fear, and anger that they hold—will always be with us, as they are our history, our legacy, and our responsibility.

But what we are seeing within Normalization is something we had not prepared for: AIDS cultural work created not in or about silence or trauma, but rather built upon connection, history, utterances of remembering and fear, and new forms of knowledge production. We are products of our own Times of AIDS. It took us time, together, to be able to see or name an AIDS present and future, being expressed now, informed but not burdened by trauma. As Alex said in an earlier draft of this conclusion, "As it turns out, there might be an afterlife to the trauma of silence."

CONCLUSION

WHAT DOES COVID-19 HAVE TO DO WITH
AIDS [CRISIS] NORMALIZATION?

In March 2020, we found ourselves in a new pandemic. As AIDS was ongoing, and ever more visible, COVID-19 emerged, Black Lives Matter protests reemerged and intensified, and the 2020 American presidential election loomed large. Unlike the early days of AIDS, when COVID-19 entered the world it seemed that everyone knew about it, everyone was afraid, and mainstream media, healthcare, and government responded. Money flowed. Research was expedited. And as part of this global and immediate attention, we noticed something else: in this context of new trauma, violence, fear, and restriction, AIDS became even more and oddly less visible.[2]

Within a short but intense period starting in 2020 (one still unfolding), a renewed interest in AIDS emerged specifically and forcefully in connection to the world's efforts to better understand COVID-19. The red-hot glare of this pandemic magnified a significant interest in AIDS culture that had already resulted from AIDS Crisis Revisitation. Citizens, academics, activists, and news anchors alike expressed new curiosity about AIDS. And in the face of another worldwide pandemic, AIDS was being seen and positioned differently.

COVID-19 put a different frame on AIDS. First of all, AIDS was suddenly less anomalous. For people far outside the world of epidemiology or HIV, COVID-19 placed AIDS into a longer narrative. In magazines, on podcasts, and in news reports AIDS was being mentioned daily, but this was in lists alongside ZIKA, H1N1, SARS, and other infectious diseases. It was understood as one among many deadly viruses from which we could learn, as well as from which we could get seriously ill.

COVID-19 also put AIDS newly into time, into history. Contemporary AIDS cultural production and COVID-19 are making clear that while no Time of AIDS is ever over, the Revisitation worked. The past of AIDS has been remembered enough that AIDS cultural production can now focus on this epidemic in the present. During COVID-19, questions about what can be learned from AIDS become newly relevant, newly useful, newly normalized. These questions are asked all the time by new (and old) communities. During COVID-19 Alex and Ted attend any number of Zoom talks, meetings, presentations, and breakout rooms about the connections between AIDS and COVID-19.

At one such event—memorable enough that Alex relayed it to Ted more than once, and then he incredulously went to watch the video recording of it to make sure it was just as bad as she said—Alex heard a respected, educated, queer of color activist intellectual introduce a panel on this very matter, featuring three other esteemed scholars of AIDS, illness, queer of color critique, and feminism. He used the phrase "the last epidemic." As in, the one before. The one that is done. The one that leads to this new one. He said this many times, but at the second iteration of this phrase, Alex piped up in the chat (having to take the bold move of being the first in this curious space). She typed, as politely as she knew how: "Of course, the AIDS pandemic is ongoing." That is, it can't be the last one, the previous one, because it is still here.

Because the esteemed professor did not see the chat as he was reading aloud his introduction into the Zoom void, he kept on referring not to AIDS, but to the "last pandemic," throughout his otherwise thoughtful introduction. It was only later that he corrected this embalming of AIDS into the past. His unintentional and short-sighted move let AIDS be in and only history, using AIDS to see today's world as a useful tool, but only temporarily. Because he self-corrected, AIDS [Crisis] Normalization allows Alex, or any of us, to engage with someone else about AIDS, confident that upon reflection people will remember what they know now: that AIDS is not over, that many Times of AIDS can and should be copresent.

RETURN: CAN YOU BRING IT? WHAT IS YOUR AIDS?

Toward the end of *Can You Bring It?* as performance-day looms, LeBlanc poses a question to the group: "What is your AIDS?" At this point in the process the dancers have overcome any limits of their bodies; they are mastering the choreography. But LeBlanc is aware that something is missing. Even as nondancers, we feel that too. Her question posed to them—What is your AIDS?—is a highly charged invitation to consider their own personal pain or struggle, one that is deep enough to fully animate their performance.

There is a given now: AIDS no longer animates.

Her question marks a strange and unanticipated acceptance that marks this Time of AIDS. These young people are not encountering AIDS as did LeBlanc, Jones, and the troupe who originally made the dance. They do not really know or fear it. Are not motivated into deep feeling, art, or power through it. After LeBlanc asks the question, the camera lingers on the young dancers' faces as they diligently and conscientiously search for an answer. They reach: The environment? Social media and feeling isolated? Cruel friends?

To the directors' credit, neither the film nor its contemporary dancers provide a resolution to this open-ended multiplicity and uncertainty that defines many contemporary AIDS experiences and art that are live in a room or troupe. In the film, the gap across generations is not erased or simplified, but neither is it total. Unlike during AIDS Crisis Revisitation, however, this difference is not a motivation for debate or distress. It looms, absent and present, different and the same, in the past and the present, as a [Crisis]. Multiple Times of AIDS can coexist and co-inform. This is hard and easy.

The performance is a success, even as the transmission of AIDS-related experiences from the past remains incomplete or perhaps unnecessary. AIDS is something the young dancers know to be true, something they are curious about and committed to, and yet they are not and cannot be traumatized by it, even as they are asked to listen to and witness Jones and LeCompte render their horrible and poignant memories, even as they enact a dance that registers this very pain. The new dancers work to honor this history, and a desire to survive and thrive that is also at the heart of the dance, even as they push themselves to feel their own pain as a place from which to hold the movement. They carry forward and embody a message that AIDS is both history and not over; theirs and others and all of ours; about pain and loss but also dance, community, and remembering.

The film ends with an ambivalence around AIDS knowledge and history that sums up this new Time we find ourselves in: with neither mass death and silence, nor history and unprocessed trauma being the dominant concern of AIDS discourse. The stakes have changed. There is perhaps a new faith that the urgencies, messages, memorials, and lessons of the previous Times of AIDS can be communicated between people and across cultures and generations and over time because they have increasingly become a normalized part of our culture, which is not to say normal. The extraordinary experience of AIDS is ongoing, and ripe with information. This is a profound benefit of Normalization amid an ever changing [Crisis].

We think that AIDS [Crisis] Normalization is unfolding, and it will take time, conversation, and community to live through and understand it. We do not know the future of AIDS, but we know that we and you will be in and of it. So this conclusion is also a beginning. Sort of like where we were when we first started conversing about the Revisitation seven years ago. We are just starting to draw connections and conclusions about Normalization; we need more time to understand this Time of AIDS.

We end this book how we started, with prompts and questions, a commitment to conversation, and an invitation to know your own Time of AIDS.

225

BEGIN THIS CONVERSATION, AGAIN

1 **LOOK AND LISTEN**

Take account of all the mentions of AIDS you encounter over a period of time that you set and now that you have read this book.

2 **CONSIDER**

Share your list with others. Do they fit well into one or more of our Times of AIDS?

3 **LOCATE**

What does this list, and your own records, reflections, and encounters made while reading this book, tell you about your own Time of AIDS?

SOURCES AND INFLUENCES TIMELINE 3

This is our creative encounter with a mediography and bibliography. It holds many of the videos, films, books, texts, exhibitions, plays, and projects that have informed our writing. This is not an exhaustive list. It is deeply personal, a highly subjective timeline of AIDS cultural production from 1981 until when we turned in our final manuscript in December 2021. It is also a self-portrait of the two of us. It captures and shares some of the work that has shaped us as individuals and as a writing duo. It holds our work, that of our friends and people we admire, as well as folks we will never know. The silences, gaps, and absences are many. For example, works of theater, dance, and poetry are sparse. We rarely include individual pieces of visual art. But within these limits there is still much room for an abundance, brilliance, and bounty of information and inspiration in which we write and learn across the Times and things of AIDS.

We make our AIDS work inside of community, alongside comrades, relying on the work of those before us, and anticipating those who will engage our work. In our communities—just as is true in this timeline—a self-awareness around ownership, legacy, authorship, and voice is paramount, and can be approached responsively. As just one example of an ample and invigorating conversation, one of our friends and colleagues, T. L. Cowan, advises that "citation is not enough":

The politics of citation—to cite down rather than up, to cite sources that are not already in massive circulation, to cite predominantly women, people of color, trans folks, Indigenous peoples, folks from the Global South, etc.—is an important form of intellectual activism meant to center the ideas of these folks rather than perpetually re-centering the ideas of mostly white, Euro-American settler dude-experts.[1]

We join this effort with this final timeline, inventing a shape to center the inspiring voices of our vast AIDS community in Times. Frankly, choosing when to stop adding to this list was harder than making it. We know it can never include all the people, art, projects, and ideas that have influenced our AIDS work.

So again: please, join us. We are having this conversation now. Dive into our third timeline. Seek patterns and relationships. Ask questions. Trouble objects that, while made in their year, seem to be in the "wrong" Time of AIDS. And jump around. But also, make note of who and what is lost. Add to our list, add your name and work, as well as those that have formed you.

1981
"Disease Rumours Largely Unfounded." Dr. Lawrence D. Mass. TEXT
"Pneumocystis Pneumonia—Los Angeles." Dr. M. S. Gottlieb. TEXT

1982
Gay Men's Health Crisis. PROJECT

1983
AIDS candlelight march. PROJECT
"The Denver Principles." Advisory committee of the People with
    AIDS. TEXT
"How to Have Sex in an Epidemic: One Approach." Michael Callen
    and Richard Berkowitz, with Dr. Joseph Sonnabend. TEXT

1985
AIDS Quilt. The NAMES Project AIDS Memorial Quilt. PROJECT
As Is. William M. Hoffman. THEATER
Bebashi. Rashidah Abdul-Khabeer and Wesley Anderson. PROJECT
Buddies. Arthur J. Bressan. FILM
The Normal Heart. Larry Kramer. THEATER

The People with AIDS Coalition. PROJECT
Sex and Germs. Cindy Patton. BOOK
Third World AIDS Advisory Task Force. Ernest Andrews, Calu Lester, and Larry Saxon. PROJECT

1986

ADODI. Clifford Rawlins. PROJECT
AIDS in the Mind of America. Dennis Altman. BOOK
Conference on Ethnic Minorities and AIDS. Third World AIDS Advisory Task Force. PROJECT
Silence = Death. The Silence = Death Project. PROJECT
Snow Job: The Media Hysteria of AIDS. Barbara Hammer. VIDEO

1987

ACT UP. PROJECT
AIDS and People of Color: The Discriminatory Impact. AIDS Discrimination Unit of New York City Commission on Human Rights. TEXT
AIDS: Keywords. Jan Zita Grover. TEXT
And the Band Played On: Politics, People, and the AIDS Epidemic. Randy Shilts. BOOK
Living with AIDS: Women and AIDS. Alexandra Juhasz and Jean Carlomusto. VIDEO
Making It! Woman's Guide to Sex in the Age of AIDS. Cindy Patton and Janis Kelly. BOOK
MIX NYC: Lesbian and Gay Experimental Film Festival. Sarah Schulman and Jim Hubbard. PROJECT
Ojos Que No Ven/Eyes That Fail to See. Jose Guitierrez-Gomez and Jose Vergelin. VIDEO
Reframing AIDS. Pratibha Parmar. VIDEO
Safe Sex Slut. Carol Leigh. VIDEO
Testing the Limits: NYC. Testing The Limits Collective. VIDEO
This Is Not an AIDS Advertisement. Isaac Julian. VIDEO
Women, Children, and AIDS. Jane Wagner. VIDEO

1988

AIDS Cultural Analysis, Cultural Activism. Douglas Crimp, ed. BOOK
AIDS: Me and My Baby. Sandra Elkin. VIDEO
AIDS: The Burdens of History. Elizabeth Fee and Daniel Fox, eds. BOOK

AIDS: The Women. Ines Rieder and Patricia Ruppelt, eds. BOOK

Blaming AIDS: Prejudice, Race, and Worldwide AIDS. Renee Sabatier. BOOK

Bleach, Teach, and Outreach. Ray Navarro and Catherine Saalfield [Gund]. VIDEO

"Bodies and Anti-Bodies: A Crisis in Representation." Timothy Landers. TEXT

Doctors, Liars, and Women. Jean Carlomusto and Maria Maggenti. VIDEO

Her Giveaway. Mona Smith. VIDEO

Latex and Lace. Laird Sutton, Janet Taylor, and Dolores Bishop. VIDEO

"Lesbian Safety and AIDS: The Very Last Fairy Tale." Lee Chiaramonte. TEXT

Mildred Pearson: When You Love a Person. Yannick Durand. VIDEO

National AIDS Memorial. PROJECT

"Needed (For Women and Children)." Suki Ports. TEXT

Prostitutes, Risk, and AIDS. Alexandra Juhasz and Jean Carlomusto. VIDEO

PWA Power. Gregg Bordowitz and Jean Carlomusto. VIDEO

Seize Control of the FDA. Gregg Bordowitz and Jean Carlomusto. VIDEO

Song from an Angel. David Weissman. VIDEO

A Test for the Nation: Women, Children, Families, AIDS. Alexandra Juhasz. VIDEO

Visual AIDS. PROJECT

Women and AIDS: A Survival Kit. VIDEO

Work Your Body: Options for People Who Are HIV-Positive. Gregg Bordowitz and Jean Carlomusto. VIDEO

1989

AIDS and the Third World. Panos Institute. BOOK

AIDS in the Barrio: Eso No Me Pasa a Mi. Frances Negron-Muntaner and Peter Biella. VIDEO

AIDS: Not Us. Harry Howard. VIDEO

AIDS: The Artists' Response. Jan Zita Grover, ed. EXHIBITION + TEXT

Are You with Me? M. Neema Barnette. VIDEO

Asian and Pacific Islander Coalition on HIV/AIDS. PROJECT

Clips. Debbie Sundhal. VIDEO

Covering the Plague: AIDS and the American Media. James Kinsella. BOOK

Critical Path AIDS Project. Kiyoshi Kuromiya. PROJECT

Current Flow. Jean Carlomusto. VIDEO

Day without Art. Visual AIDS. PROJECT

DHPG Mon Amour. Carl Michael George. VIDEO

DiAna's Hair Ego: AIDS Info UpFront. Ellen Spiro. VIDEO
"Do It!" Gregg Bordowitz and Jean Carlmuto. TEXT
"Dynamics of Black Mobilization against AIDS in New York City."
　　Ernest Quimby and Samuel R. Friedman. TEXT
Elegy in the Streets. Jim Hubbard. VIDEO
He Left Me His Strength. Sherry Busbee. VIDEO
The Irreversible Decline of Eddie Socket. John Weir. BOOK
"Mourning and Militancy." Douglas Crimp. TEXT
"Not Just Black and White: AIDS Media and People of Color." Ray Na-
　　varro and Catherine Saalfield [Gund]. TEXT
Pediatric AIDS: A Time of Crisis. Pierce Atkins. VIDEO
Safer Sex Shorts. Multiple directors, GMHC. VIDEO
The Second Epidemic. Amber Hollibaugh. VIDEO
"Seeing through AIDS." Media Network. TEXT
Se Met Ko. Patritia Benoit. VIDEO
Seriously Fresh. Reggie Life. VIDEO
"Sexuality: Reproductive Technologies and AIDS." Elizabeth Weed and
　　Naomi Schor, eds. In *differences: Special Issue on Life Death*. TEXT
Taking Liberties. Erica Carter and Simon Watney, eds. BOOK
Target City Hall. DIVA TV. VIDEO
This Is a Dental Dam. Suzanne Wright. VIDEO
Tongues Untied. Marlon Riggs. VIDEO
Untitled. John Sanborn. VIDEO
Vida. Lourdes Portillo. VIDEO
Viva Eu! Tania Cypriano. VIDEO
With Loving Arms. Children's Welfare League of America. VIDEO

1990

AIDS Demographics. Douglas Crimp. BOOK
(An) Other Love Story: Women and AIDS. Gabrielle Micallef and Debbie
　　Douglas. VIDEO Between Friends. Severo Perez. VIDEO
Angels in America. Tony Kushner. THEATER
Caring for Infants and Toddlers with HIV Infection. Children's Welfare
　　League of America. VIDEO
"Diseased Pariah News." Beowulf Thorne, Tom Shearer, Tom Ace, and
　　Michael Botkin. PROJECT
Ecstatic Antibodies: Resisting the AIDS Mythology. Sunil Gupta and Tessa
　　Boffin, eds. BOOK
El Abrazo (The Embrace). Diana Coryat. VIDEO
Fear of Disclosure. Phil Zwicker and David Wojnarowicz. VIDEO
Fighting Chance. Richard Fung. VIDEO

Fighting for Our Lives. Center for Women's Policy Studies. VIDEO
The Forgotten People: Latinas with AIDS. Hector Galan. VIDEO
Inventing AIDS. Cindy Patton. BOOK
Karate Kids. Derek Lamb. VIDEO
Keep Your Laws Off My Body. Catherine Saalfield [Gund] and Zoe Leonard. VIDEO
Kissing Doesn't Kill. Gran Fury. VIDEO
Mi Hermano. Edgar Michael Bravo. VIDEO.
"Minority Women and AIDS." Dooley Worth. TEXT
People in Trouble. Sarah Schulman. BOOK
So Sad, So Sorry, So What. Jane Gillooly. VIDEO
Speak for Yourself. Jim Hubbard. VIDEO
Steam Clean. Richard Fung. VIDEO
Stop the Church. Richard Hillferty. VIDEO
"Strategic Compromises: AIDS and Alternative Video Practices." John Greyson. TEXT
Too Close for Comfort. Peg Cambell. VIDEO
To the Friend Who Did Not Save My Life. Hervé Guibert. BOOK
A WAVE Taster. Women's AIDS Video Enterprise. VIDEO
We Care: A Video for Care Providers of People Affected by AIDS. WAVE (Women's AIDS Video Enterprise). VIDEO
Women, AIDS & Activism. The ACT UP/ NY Women & AIDS Book Group. BOOK

1991
Absolutely Positive. Peter Adair. VIDEO
BOLO! BOLO! Gita Saxena and Ian Rashid. VIDEO
Close to the Knives: A Memoir of Disintegration. David Wojnarowicz. BOOK
"The Ethics of Community Media: A Filmmaker Confronts the Contradictions of Producing Media about and for a Community Where She Is Both Insider and Outsider." Frances Negron-Muntaner. TEXT
Fighting in Southwest Louisiana. Peter Friedman. VIDEO
Hard to Get. Alisa Lebow. VIDEO
Identities. Nino Rodriquez. VIDEO
(in)Visible Women. Marna Alvarez and Ellen Spiro. VIDEO
It's Not Easy. Faustin J. Misanvu. VIDEO
Like a Prayer. DIVA TV. VIDEO
Native Americans, Two Spirits and HIV. Indian Community House. VIDEO
"Outlaws through the Lens of Corporate America." Ellen Spiro. TEXT

Prowling by Night. Gwendolyn. VIDEO
Thinking about Death. Gregg Bordowitz. VIDEO
Two Marches. Jim Hubbard. VIDEO
"Video, AIDS, and Activism." Ann Cvetovich. TEXT

1992

Acting Up for Prisoners. Eric Slade and Mic Sweeney. VIDEO
ACT TV Public Access Series. James Wentzy (1992–1994). PROJECT
AIDS and Accusation: Haiti and the Geography of Blame. Paul Farmer.
   BOOK
AIDS Is About Secrets. Sandra Elkin. VIDEO
AIDS: Life at Stake. Heather E. Edmondson. VIDEO
AIDS: The Making of a Chronic Disease. Elizabeth Fox and Daniel Fee,
   eds. BOOK
Belinda. Anne Lewis Johnson. VIDEO
Ceremonies. Essex Hemphill. BOOK
Condomnation. Anne Chamberlain. VIDEO
I'm You, You're Me: Women Surviving Prison, Living with AIDS. Debra
   Levine and Catherine Saafield [Gund]. VIDEO
Kecia. Peter Von Puttkamer. VIDEO.
A Leap in the Dark. Allan Klusacek and Ken Morrison, eds. BOOK
Le Ravissement. Charline Boudreau. VIDEO
My Body's My Business. Vivian Kleinman. VIDEO
Non, Je Ne Regrette Rien (No Regret). Marlon Riggs. VIDEO
No Rewind: Teenagers Speak Out on HIV/AIDS Awareness. Paula Mozen.
   VIDEO
Party Safe! with Bambi and DiAna. Ellen Spiro. VIDEO
Pitimi San Gado (Millet Without a Guardian). Hatian Teens Confront
   AIDS. VIDEO
Positive Women: Voices of Women Living with AIDS. Andrea Rudd and
   Darien Taylor, eds. BOOK
SafeSister. Maria Perez and Wellington Love. VIDEO
Simple Courage: An Historical Portrait for the Age of AIDS. Stephanie Cas-
   tillo. VIDEO
Voices from the Front. Testing the Limits Collective. VIDEO
Voices of Positive Women. Darien Taylor and Michael Balser. VIDEO
Was. Geoff Ryman. BOOK

1993

Caring Segments. Juanita Mohammed (Szczepanski). VIDEO
The Faces of AIDS. Frances Reid. VIDEO

Fluid Exchanges: Artists and Critics in the AIDS Crisis. James Miller, ed.
BOOK
Grid-Lock: Women and the Politics of AIDS. Beth Wichterich. VIDEO
Heart of the Matter. Gini Retticker and Amber Hollibaugh. FILM
It Is What It Is . . . Gregg Bordowitz. VIDEO
"Notes on AIDS and Its Combatants: An Appreciation." Bill Horrigan.
TEXT
*One Foot on a Banana Peel, the Other Foot in the Grave (Secrets from the
Dolly Madison Room).* Juan Botas and Lucas Platt. VIDEO
Part of Me. Juanita Mohammed (Szczepanski) and Alisa Lebow. VIDEO
Party! Charles Sessoms. VIDEO
Philadelphia. Jonathan Demme. FILM
Positively Women. Nalini Singh. VIDEO
Reunion. Jamal Joseph and Laverne Berry. VIDEO
Safe Is Desire. Debi Sundhal. VIDEO
Safe Love. Lori Ayers, Eric N. Duran, and Ellen V. Shapiro. VIDEO
Safer and Sexier: A College Student's Guide to Safer Sex. The Lay Techs Ed-
ucation Group. VIDEO
Silverlake Life: The View from Here. Tom Joslin and Peter Friedman. FILM
Women and AIDS: Psychological Perspectives. Corinne Squire, ed. BOOK
Writing AIDS. Timothy Murphy and Suzanne Poirier, eds. BOOK
Zero Patience. John Greyson. FILM

1994

"Against the Law: Sex Workers Speak." Cynthia Chris. TEXT
Fast Trip, Long Drop. Gregg Bordowitz. FILM
My American History: Lesbian and Gay Life during the Reagan/Bush Years.
Sarah Schulman. BOOK
Practices of Freedom: Selected Writings on HIV/AIDS. Simon Watney. BOOK
Rent. Jonathan Larson. THEATER

1995

AIDS TV. Alexandra Juhasz. BOOK
In the Shadow of the Epidemic. Walt Odets. BOOK

1996

At Odds with AIDS: Thinking and Talking about a Virus. Alexander García
Düttmann. BOOK
The Body of this Death: Historicity and Sociality in the Time of AIDS. Wil-
liam Wendell Haver. BOOK

Fatal Advice: How Safe-Sex Education Went Wrong. Cindy Patton. BOOK
Gary in Your Pocket. Gary Fisher. BOOK
HIV: Un-infected Un-affected. David Weissman. FILM
"When Plagues End." Andrew Sullivan. TEXT

1997

Killing the Black Body. Dorothy Roberts. BOOK
"Punks, Bulldaggers, and Welfare Queens: The Radical Potential of
     Queer Politics?" Cathy J. Cohen. TEXT
RePlacing Citizenship: AIDS Activism and Radical Democracy. Michael P.
     Brown. BOOK
*Tangled Memories: The Vietnam War, the AIDS Epidemic, and the Politics of
     Remembering*. Marita Sturken. BOOK
Two Men and a Baby. Juanita Mohammed (Szczepanski). VIDEO
Unbecoming. Eric Michaels. BOOK

1998

Acts of Intervention: Performance, Gay Culture, and AIDS. David Roman.
     BOOK
Blind Eye to Justice. Carol Leigh. VIDEO
*Breaking the Fine Rain of Death: African American Health Issues and a Wom-
     anist Ethic of Care*. Emilie Townes. BOOK
*Breaking the Walls of Silence: AIDS and Women in a New York State Maximum
     Security Prison*. ACE (AIDS Counseling and Education Program).
     BOOK
*Breaking the Walls of Silence: AIDS and Women in a New York State Maximum
     Security Prison*. Kathy Boudin, ed. BOOK
Dry Bones Breathe: Gay Men Creating Post-AIDS Identities and Cultures. Eric
     Rofes. BOOK
Koolaids: The Art of War. Rabih Alameddine. BOOK
Stagestruck. Sarah Schulman. BOOK

1999

The Blackwater Lightship. Colm Tóibín. BOOK
The Boundaries of Blackness: AIDS and the Breakdown of Black Politics. Cathy
     Cohen. BOOK
Christ Like. Emanuel Xavier. BOOK
How to Have Theory in an Epidemic: The Cultural Chronicle of AIDS. Paula
     Treichler. BOOK

2000

Representations of HIV and AIDS: Visibility Blue/s. Gabriele Griffin. BOOK
Shatzi Is Dying. Jean Carlomusto. VIDEO

2001

Negative Thoughts. AA Bronson. BOOK

2002

ACT UP Oral History Project. Sarah Schulman and Jim Hubbard, with
camerawork by James Wentzy, S. Leo Chiang, and Tracy Ware.
PROJECT
AIDS Activist Videotape Collection, 1983–2000. New York Public Li-
brary Humanities and Social Sciences Library Manuscripts and
Archives Division. Jim Hubbard. PROJECT
"Critical Investments: AIDS, Christopher Reeve, and Queer/Disability
Studies." Robert McRuer. TEXT
Fight Back, Fight AIDS: 15 Years of ACT UP. James Wentzy. VIDEO
Melancholia and Moralism: Essays on AIDS and Queer Politics. Douglas
Crimp. BOOK
*Outlaw Representation: Censorship and Homosexuality in Twentieth-Century
Art.* Richard Meyer. BOOK
Publics and Counterpublics. Michael Warner. BOOK

2003

An Archive of Feelings. Anne Cvetkovich. BOOK
Corpus Magazine. George Ayala, Jaime Cortez and Pato Hebert.
PROJECT
PEPFAR. United States Government. PROGRAM
Pills Profits Protest. Shanti Avirgan, Anne-Christine D'Adesky and Ann
T. Rossetti. FILM
Queer Latinidad: Identity Practices, Discursive Spaces. Juana Maria Rodri-
guez. BOOK

2004

The AIDS Crisis Is Ridiculous and Other Writings: 1986–2003. Gregg
Bordowitz. BOOK
*How to Make Dances in an Epidemic: Tracking Choreography in the Age of
AIDS.* David Gere. BOOK
Los Nutcrackers: A Christmas Carajo. Charles Rice-González. THEATER

Notorious H.I.V.: The Media Spectacle of Nushawn Williams. Thomas
    Shevory. BOOK
When AIDS Began: San Francisco and the Making of an Epidemic. Michelle
    Cochrane. BOOK
*Workable Sisterhood: The Political Journey of Stigmatized Women with
    HIV/AIDS.* Michele Tracy Berger. BOOK
Writing AIDS. Sarah Brophy. BOOK

2005
Veronica. Mary Gaitskill. BOOK
Video Remains. Alexandra Juhasz. VIDEO

2006
"Retroactivism." Lucas Hilderbrand. TEXT
"Video Remains: Nostalgia, Technology, and Queer Archive Activ-
    ism." Alexandra Juhasz. TEXT

2007
Life Support. Nelson George. VIDEO
Treatments: Language, Politics, and the Culture of Illness. Lisa Diedrich.
    BOOK
Where Did the Love Go? Nelson Santos, featuring Nayland Blake,
    Erik Hanson, Lou Laurita, and Nancer LeMoins. PROJECT

2008
Another Planet. Stefano Tummolini. VIDEO
Chronicle of a Plague, Revisited: AIDS and Its Aftermath. Andrew Holleran.
    BOOK
The Invisible Cure. Helen Epstein. BOOK
Me Mengwa Maa Sinatae: Butterfly Patterns of Light. Marjorie Beaucage.
    VIDEO
Pedro. Nick Oceano. VIDEO
Sex Positive. Daryl Wein. FILM
"The Swiss Statement." Swiss National AIDS Commission. TEXT
Wild Combination: A Portrait of Arthur Russell. Matt Wolf. FILM
Wish You Were Here: Memories of a Gay Life. Sunil Gupta. BOOK

2009

ACT UP New York: Activism, Art, and the AIDS Crisis, 1987–1993. Helen
    Molesworth and Claire Grace. EXHIBITION
"Against Equality, in Maine and Everywhere." Ryan Conrad. TEXT
Boundaries of Contagion: How Ethnic Politics Have Shaped Government Re-
    sponses to AIDS. Evan S. Lieberman. BOOK
Cruising Utopia: The Then and There of Queer Futurity. Jose Muñoz. BOOK
Fig Trees. John Greyson. FILM
Infectious Ideas: U.S. Political Responses to the AIDS Crisis. Jennifer Brier.
    BOOK
Moving Politics: Emotion and ACT UP's Fight against AIDS. Deborah Gould.
    BOOK
Precious. Lee Daniels. FILM
Reframing Bodies: AIDS, Bearing Witness, and the Queer Moving Image.
    Roger Hallas. BOOK
Sex in an Epidemic. Jean Carlomusto. FILM
Virus Alert: Security, Governmentality, and the AIDS Pandemic. Stefan Elbe.
    BOOK
The Wisdom of Whores: Bureaucrats, Brothels, and the Business of AIDS. Eliz-
    abeth Pisani. BOOK

2010

"Contagious: Cultures, Carriers, and the Outbreak Narrative." Pris-
    cilla Wald. TEXT
For Colored Girls. Tyler Perry. FILM
General Idea: Image Virus. Gregg Bordowitz. BOOK
Hide/Seek: Difference and Desire in American Portraiture. Jonathan Katz
    and David C. Ward. EXHIBITION
Last Address. Ira Sachs. VIDEO
"Moving Pictures: AIDS on Film and Video." Debra Levine. TEXT
QUEEROCRACY. Michael Tikili, Megan Mulholland, Camilo Godoy,
    and Cassidy Gardner. PROJECT
Red Red Red. David Oscar Harvey. VIDEO

2011

Digital Stories. Margaret Rhee, Isela Ford, and Allyse Gray. VIDEO
Heart Breaks Open. William Maria Rain. FILM
he said. Irwin Swirnoff. VIDEO
HIV Is Not a Crime. Sean Strub. VIDEO
If Memory Serves. Chris Castiglia and Chris Reed. BOOK
Inside Lara Roxx. Mia Donovan. FILM

Inside Story. Rolie Nikiwe. FILM
Liberaceón. Chris Vargas. VIDEO
Life above All. Oliver Schmitz. FILM
PosterVirus. Alexander McClelland and Jessica Whitbread for AIDS
    ACTION NOW! PROJECT
Queer Retrosexualities: The Politics of Reparative Return. Nishant Shahani.
    BOOK
30 Years from Here. Josh Rosenzweig. FILM
Untitled. Jim Hodges, Carlos Marques da Cruz, and Encke King.
    VIDEO
Vito. Jeffrey Schwarz. FILM
We Were Here. David Weisman. FILM

2012
"ACT UP, Haitian Migrants, and Alternative Memories of HIV/ AIDS."
    Karma R. Chavez. TEXT
"ACT UP in Film: How to Survive a Plague and United in Anger."
    Simon Collins. TEXT
"AIDS at a Nexus." Philip Kennicott. TEXT
"AIDS 2.0." Avram Finkelstein. TEXT
The Already Dead: The New Time of Politics, Culture, and Illness. Eric
    Cazdyn. BOOK
Black Bodies and the Black Church: A Blues Slant. Kelly Brown Douglas.
    BOOK
Bumming Cigarettes. Tiona McClodden. VIDEO
Carlos Motta: We Who Feel Differently. Eungie Joo. EXHIBITION
Coming After. Jon Davis. TEXT + EXHIBITION
Ending Silence, Shame, Stigma: HIV/AIDS in the African American Family.
    Katherine Cheairs. VIDEO
Fire in the Belly: The Life and Times of David Wojnarowicz. Cynthia Carr.
    BOOK
"Forgetting ACT UP." Alexandra Juhasz. TEXT
Gentrification of the Mind. Sarah Schulman. BOOK
Gran Fury: Read My Lips. Gran Fury and Michael Cohen. EXHIBITION
Haute Culture: General Idea. Frédéric Bonne. EXHIBITION
How to Survive a Plague. David France. FILM
I Always Said Yes. Jim Tushinski. FILM
"I'm Not the Man I Used to Be: Sex, HIV, and Cultural 'Responsibil-
    ity.'" Christopher M. Bell. TEXT
Keep the Lights On. Ira Sachs. FILM
Last Address Tribute Walk. Alex Fialho. PROJECT

Positive Women: Exposing Injustice. Alison Duke. VIDEO

"The Proximate Truth: Reenactment in the Pandemic-Era HIV/AIDS Documentaries." Bishnupriya Ghosh. TEXT

"Reflecting on ACT UP . . . Honestly." Sean Strub. TEXT

This Will Have Been: Art, Love & Politics in the 1980s. Helen Molesworth. TEXT + EXHIBITION

Tinderbox: How the West Sparked the AIDS Epidemic and How the World Can Finally Overcome It. Craig Timberg and Daniel Halperin. BOOK

Toxic Beauty: The Art of Frank Moore. Susan Harris with Lynn Gumpert. EXHIBITION

"Truvada Whores?" David Duran. TEXT

United in Anger: A History of ACT UP. Jim Hubbard. FILM

Viral. Patricia Clough and Jasbir Puar, eds. BOOK

2013

AIDS in New York: The First Five Years. Jean Ashton. EXHIBITION

The Battle of AmfAR. Rob Epstein and Jeffrey Friedman. FILM

"Becoming-Undetectable." Nathan Lee. TEXT

Behind the Candelabra. Steven Soderbergh. FILM

Dallas Buyers Club. Jean-Marc Vallée. FILM

Fairyland: A Memoir of My Father. Alysia Abbott. BOOK

Fire in the Blood. Dylan Mohan Gray. FILM

For the Record. fierce pussy. PROJECT

"Ghost Stories." David Oscar Harvey, Marty Fink, Alexandra Juhasz, and Bishnu Gosh. TEXT

"Haunting the Queer Spaces of AIDS: Remembering ACT UP/NY and an Ethics of an Epidemic." Julian Gill-Peterson. TEXT

"How to Whitewash a Plague." Hugh Ryan. TEXT

I Loved You More. Tom Spanbauer. BOOK

I, You, We. David Kiehl. EXHIBITION

Let The Record Show. Demetrea Dewald. FILM

NOT OVER: 25 Years of Visual AIDS. Sur Rodney Sur, and Kris Nuzzi. EXHIBITION

NYC 1993: Experimental Jet Set, Trash and No Star. Massimiliano Gioni, Gary Carrion-Murayari, Jenny Moore, and Margot Norton. EXHIBITION

Philomena. Stephen Frears. FILM

"(re)Presenting AIDS in Public." Visual AIDS. TEXT

Revisiting the AIDS Crisis: A Conversation with David France and Jim Hubbard. The New School and Visual AIDS. EVENT + VIDEO

Safe Sex Bang: The Buzz Bense Collection of Safe Sex Posters. Alex Fialho and Dorian Katz. TEXT + EXHIBITION

Safe Space: Gay Neighborhood History and the Politics of Violence. Christina B. Hanhardt. BOOK

Short Memory/No History. Jack Waters and Peter Cramer. VIDEO + PROJECT

Structural Intimacies: Sexual Stories in the Black AIDS Epidemic. Sonja Mackenzie. BOOK

Temptation. Tyler Perry. FILM

The Test. Chris Mason Johnson. FILM

They Glow in the Dark. Panayotis Evangelidis. FILM

Things are Different Now . . . Ryan Conrad. VIDEO

When Did You Figure Out You Had AIDS? Vincent Chevalier. VIDEO

Why We Fight: Remembering AIDS Activism. Jason Baumann and Laura Karas. EXHIBITION

2014

About [insert] boy. Danez Smith. BOOK

Against Equality: Queer Revolution, Not Mere Inclusion. Ryan Conrad, ed. BOOK

Age of Consent. Todd Verow and Charles Lum. VIDEO

All Yours. David Lambert. FILM

Antiblack Racism and the AIDS Epidemic: State Intimacies. Adam M. Geary. BOOK

Ashes. Tom Kalin. VIDEO

Back on Board: Greg Louganis. Cheryl Furjanic. FILM

Black Gay Genius: Answering Joseph Beam's Call. Charles Stephens & Steven G. Fullwood. BOOK

Body Counts: A Memoir of Politics, Sex, AIDS, and Survival. Sean Strub. BOOK

Califórnia. Marina Person. FILM

The Counter Narrative Project. Charles Stephens. PROJECT

Counterpublicity. My Barbarian. VIDEO

Dear Lou Sullivan. Rhys Ernst. VIDEO

evidence. Julie Tolentino and Abigail Severance. VIDEO

The Gran Varones. Louie A. Ortiz-Fonseca. PROJECT

Hold Tight Gently: Michael Callen, Essex Hemphill, and the Battlefield of AIDS. Martin Duberman. BOOK

Keith Haring: The Political Line. Dieter Buchhart. TEXT + EXHIBITION

The Nearness of Others: Searching for Tact and Contact in the Age of HIV. David Caron. BOOK

No Easy Walk to Freedom. Nancy Nicol. FILM

The Normal Heart. Ryan Murphy. FILM

On Immunity: An Inoculation. Eula Biss. BOOK

Presente! The Ongoing Story of Latino AIDS Activism in NYC. Julian De Mayo. PROJECT

Pride. Matthew Warchus. FILM

Rebels Rebel: AIDS, Art and Activism in New York, 1979-1989. Tommaso Speretta. BOOK

7 Years Later. Glen Fogel. VIDEO

"Time Is Not a Line: Conversations, Essays, and Images about HIV/ AIDS Now." Theodore (ted) Kerr, ed. TEXT

The Village. Hi Tiger. VIDEO

"We Will Not Rest in Peace: AIDS Activism, Black Radicalism, Queer and/or Trans Resistance." Che Gossett. TEXT

"What You Don't Know About AIDS Could Fill a Museum." Visual AIDS. TEXT.

"Why I Am a Truvada Whore." Christopher Glazek. TEXT

2015

After Silence. Avram Finkelstein. BOOK

After the Wrath of God: AIDS, Sexuality, and American Religion. Anthony Michael Petro. BOOK

AIDS. Based on a True Story. Vladimir Čajkovac. EXHIBITION

Art AIDS America. Jonathan Katz and Rock Hushka, eds. BOOK + EXHIBITION

"A Black Body on Trial: The Conviction of HIV-Positive 'Tiger Mandingo.'" Steven Thrasher. TEXT

The Calendar of Loss: Race, Sexuality, and Mourning in the Early Era of AIDS. Dagmawi Woubshet. BOOK

The Chimp and the River: How AIDS Emerged from an African Forest. David Quammen. BOOK

Consent: HIV Non-Disclosure and Sexual Assault Law. Alison Duke, 2015. VIDEO

Desert Migration. Daniel Cardone, 2015. FILM

Dying Words: The AIDS Reporting of Jeff Schmalz and How It Transformed the New York Times. Samuel G. Freedman and Kerry Donahue. BOOK

"Feminists Should Recognize that HIV Criminalization Harms Women." Victoria Law. TEXT

HIV Exceptionalism: Development Through Disease in Sierra Leone. Adia Benton. BOOK

"How to Survive a Footnote: AIDS Activism in the 'After' Years." Emily Bass. TEXT

I'm Still Surviving: A Living Women's History of HIV/AIDS. Jennifer
    Brier + History Moves. PROJECT
Inflamed: A Litany for Burning Condoms. Christopher Jones, L. J. Roberts,
    Niknaz, and Theodore Kerr. VIDEO
Larry Kramer in Love and Anger. Jean Carlomusto. FILM
Last Men Standing. Erin Brethauer and Tim Hussin. FILM
Mobilizing New York: AIDS, Antipoverty and Feminist Activism. Tamar
    Caroll. BOOK
The Recollectors. Alysia Abbott and Whitney Joiner. PROJECT
Seed Money: The Chuck Holmes Story. Michael Stabile. FILM
"Sexual Pleasure as a Problem for HIV Biomedical Prevention." Kane
    Race. TEXT
Straight Outta Compton. F. Gary Gray. FILM
"Under the Rainbow." Tyrone Palmer. TEXT
Villanelle. Hayat Hyatt. VIDEO
Visions and Revisions: Coming of Age in the Age of AIDS. Dale Peck. BOOK

2016
The AIDS Memorial on Instagram. Stuart Armstrong. PROJECT
"AIDS 1969: HIV, History, and Race." Theodore (ted) Kerr. TEXT
The Angel of History. Rabih Alameddine. BOOK
À *VANCOUVER*. Vincent Chevalier. VIDEO
"Black Gay (Raw) Sex." Marlon M. Bailey. TEXT
Christodora. Tim Murphy. BOOK
"Claiming Sexual Autonomy for People with HIV through Collective
    Action." Jessica Whitbread and Alexander McClelland.
    TEXT
Compulsive Practice. Jean Carlomusto, Alexandra Juhasz, and Hugh
    Ryan. VIDEO
Everyday. Jean Carlomusto, Alexandra Juhasz, and Hugh Ryan.
    EXHIBITION
Holding the Man. Neil Armfield. FILM
"How to Survive: AIDS and Its Afterlives in Popular Media." Jih-Fei
    Cheng. TEXT
"How to Survive the Whitewashing of AIDS: Global Pasts, Transna-
    tional Futures." Nishant Shahani. TEXT
*Indian Blood: HIV and Colonial Trauma in San Francisco's Two-Spirit Com-
    munity*. Andrew Jolivette. BOOK
"Infected Sunset, Demian DinéYazhi'." TEXT
In the City of Shy Hunters. Tom Spanbauer. BOOK
It's Only the End of the World. Xavier Dolan. FILM

Lavender and Red: Liberation and Solidarity in the Gay and Lesbian Left.
Emily K. Hobson. BOOK
Lost & Found: Dance, New York, HIV/AIDS, Then and Now. Ishmael
Houston-Jones, Will Rawls, and Jaime Shearn Coan, eds. TEXT
Memories of a Penitent Heart. Cecilia Aldarondo. FILM
Paris 05:59: Théo & Hugo. Olivier Ducastel and Jacques Martineau. FILM
Positive. Linus Ignatius. VIDEO.
Pushing Dead. Tom E. Brown. FILM
Strike a Pose. Reijer Zwaan and Ester Gould. FILM
Uncle Howard. Aaron Brookner. FILM
Undetectable = Untransmittable. Prevention Access Campaign.
PROJECT
Visual Arts and the AIDS Epidemic: An Oral History Project. Archives
of American Art, Smithsonian Institution. PROJECT
Who's Gonna Love Me Now? Barak Heymann, Tomer Heymann, Alexan-
der Bodin, and Saphir. FILM
Wilhemina's War. June Cross. FILM

2017

About Face: The Evolution of a Black Producer. Thomas Allen Harris.
VIDEO
After Louie. Vincent Gagliostro. FILM
AIDS at Home: Art and Everyday Activism. Stephen Vider. EXHIBITION
"America's Hidden H.I.V. Epidemic." Linda Villarosa. TEXT
Atlantic Is a Sea of Bones. Tourmaline. VIDEO
Bending the Arc. Pedro Kos and Kief Davidson. FILM
BPM. Robin Campillo. FILM
The Death and Life of Marsha P. Johnson. David France. FILM
DiAna's Hair Ego REMIX. Cheryl Dunye & Ellen Spiro. VIDEO
Goodnight Kia. Kia LaBeija. VIDEO
"Interchange: HIV/AIDS and U.S. History." Jonathan Bell, Darius Bost,
Jennifer Brier, Julio Capo Jr., Jih-Fei Cheng, Daniel M. Fox, Chris-
tina Hanhardt, Emily Hobson, and Dan Royles. TEXT
Johnny Would You Love Me If My Dick Were Bigger? Brontez Purnell.
BOOK
The Labyrinth 1.0. Tiona Nekkia McClodden. VIDEO
*The Life and Death of ACT UP/LA: Anti-AIDS Activism in Los Angeles from
the 1980s to the 2000s*. Benita Roth. BOOK
Nothing without Us: The Women Who Will End AIDS. Harriet Hirshorn.
FILM
One Day This Kid Will Get Larger. Danny Orendorff. EXHIBITION

100 Boyfriends Mixtape (The Demo). Brontez Purnell. VIDEO
Patient Zero and the Making of the AIDS Epidemic. Richard A. McKay.
    BOOK
The Pox Lover: An Activist's Decade in New York and Paris. Anne-Christine
    d'Adesky. BOOK
PrEPahHontoz. Sheldon Raymore. PROJECT
Punishing Disease: HIV and the Criminalization of Sickness. Trevor Hoppe.
    BOOK
Selections from the Ektachrome Archive. Lyle Ashton Harris. VIDEO +
    BOOK
Silence Is a Falling Body, Augustina Comedia, FILM
Stones & Water Weight. Mykki Blanco. VIDEO
Summer 1993. Carla Simón. FILM
"Your Nostalgia Is Killing Me: Activism, Affect and the Archives of
    HIV/AIDS." Marika Cifor. TEXT

2018
ACT UP NY, for Alternate Endings, Activist Risings. ACT UP. VIDEO
After Silence: A History of AIDS through Its Images. Avram, Finkelstein.
    BOOK
"Art AIDS America Chicago." Staci Boris. TEXT
Before AIDS: Gay Health Politics in the 1970s. Katie Batza. BOOK
Bohemian Rhapsody. Bryan Singer. FILM
Cell Count. Kyle Croft and Asher Mones for Visual AIDS, EXHIBITION
    + TEXT
David Wojnarowicz: History Keeps Me Awake at Night. David Breslin and
    David W. Kiehl. TEXT
5B. Paul Haggis and Dan Krauss. FILM
The Great Believers. Rebecca Makkai. BOOK
"Grindr of Gears: An App for the Surveillance State." Abdul-Aliy Mu-
    hammad. TEXT
Happy Birthday Marsha! Reina Gossett and Sasha Wortzel. VIDEO
The HIV Howler. Jessica Whitbread and Anthea Black. PROJECT
The Library Book. Susan Orlean. BOOK
Neptune. Timothy DuWhite. THEATER
1985. Yen Tan. FILM
Nurses on the Inside: Stories of the HIV/AIDS Epidemic in NYC. Ellen Matzer
    and Valery Hughes. BOOK
A Piece of Me with HIV. Shyronn Jones. BOOK
A Place in the City: Three Stories about AIDS at Home. Nate Lavey and Ste-
    phen Vider. VIDEO

Positive Images: Gay Men and HIV/AIDS *in the Culture of "Post Crisis."* Dion Kagan. BOOK

Positive Women's Network USA, for Alternate Endings, Activist Risings. PWN-USA. VIDEO

Quiet Heroes. Jenny Mackenzie, Jared Ruga and Amanda Stoddard. FILM

Sero Project, for Alternate Endings, Activist Risings. Sero. VIDEO

Sketchtasy. Mattilda Bernstein Sycamore. BOOK

Sorry Angel. Christophe Honoré. FILM

The Spot, for Alternate Endings, Activist Risings. The Spot. VIDEO

Tacoma Action Collective, for Alternate Endings, Activist Risings. TAC. VIDEO

Vocal-NY, for Alternate Endings, Activist Risings. Vocal-NY. VIDEO

2019

"AIDS, Black Feminisms, and the Institutionalization of Queer Politics." Jih-Fei Cheng. TEXT

Archiving an Epidemic: Art, AIDS, and the Queer Chicanx Avant-Garde. Robb Hernández. BOOK

Art AIDS America Chicago. Staci Boris and Lucia Marquand. TEXT

Beat Goes On. Shanti Avirgan. VIDEO

Chloe Dzubilo: There is a Transolution. Viva Ruiz. VIDEO

Cruising the Dead River: David Wojnarowicz and New York's Ruined Waterfront. Fiona Anderson. BOOK

(ES)tatus: Reclamando el legado del Latina/o Caucus de ACT UP NY. Julian de Mayo. EXHIBITION

Evidence of Being: The Black Gay Cultural Renaissance and the Politics of Violence. Darius Bost. BOOK

(eye/virus). Jack Waters and Victor F. M. Torres. VIDEO

The Gospel of Eureka. Michael Palmieri and Donal Mosher. VIDEO

I'm Still Me. Iman Shervington. VIDEO

Inheritance (The), Matthew Lopez. THEATER

I Remember Dancing. Nguyen Tan Hoang. VIDEO

The Lie. Carl George. VIDEO

Metanoia: Transformation through AIDS Archives and Activism. Katherine Cheairs, Alexandra Juhasz, Theodore Kerr, and Jawanza Williams, eds. TEXT + EXHIBITION

Much Handled Things Are Always Soft. Derrick Woods-Morrow. VIDEO

one in two, Donja Love. THEATER

Original Plumbing: The Best of Ten Years of Trans Male Culture. Amos Mac and Rocco Kayiatos, eds. BOOK

Out of the Shadows: Reimagining Gay Men's Lives. Walt Odets. BOOK

Remaking a Life: How Women Living with HIV/AIDS Confront Inequality. Celeste Watkins-Hayes. BOOK

The Tradition. Jericho Brown. BOOK

United by AIDS: An Anthology on Art in Response to HIV/AIDS. Raphael Gygax and Heike Munder, eds. TEXT

What You Don't Know about AIDS Could Fill a Museum. Theodore (ted) Kerr, ed. BOOK

The Whole World Is Watching. J Triangular. VIDEO

2020

AIDS and the Distribution of Crises. Jih-Fei Cheng, Alexandra Juhasz, and Nishant Shahani, eds. BOOK

All the Young Men. Ruth Coker Burks. BOOK

The Big Disease with the Little Name. Maria Denise Yala. PROJECT

Can You Bring It? Bill T. Jones and D-Man in the Waters, Rosalynde LeBland and Tom Hurwitz. FILM

Can You Save Superman? Jordan Eagles. PROJECT

Female Disappearance Syndrome. Lucia Egaña Rojas. VIDEO

Final Transmission, Performance Art, and AIDS in Los Angeles. Brian Getnick and Tanya Rubbak, eds. BOOK

Finding Purpose. George Stanley Nsamba. VIDEO

The Freezer Door. Mattilda Bernstein Sycamore. BOOK

Funeral Diva. Pamela Sneed. BOOK

HIV/AIDS and Digital Media. Marika Cifor and Cait McKinney, eds. TEXT

"How to Live with a Virus." Theodore (ted) Kerr. TEXT

"In Our Bodies: A Zine about Pleasure, Intimacy, and Reality in 2020." What Would an HIV Doula Do? TEXT

Information Activism. Cait McKinney. BOOK

Keith Haring's Line: Race and the Performance of Desire. Ricardo Montez. BOOK

Lifelines. Eric Rhein. BOOK

Me Cuido. Las Indetectables. VIDEO

Ministry of Health. Jorge Bordello. VIDEO

"Our COVID-19 Response Is Living in the House HIV Activists Built." Abdul-Aliy A Muhammad. TEXT

Plague Years: A Doctor's Journey through the AIDS Crisis. Ross A. Slotten, MD. BOOK

See You There: Making History at Whitman-Walker. Ruth Noack. EXHIBITION

"Self-Reflections in 2020." Brian Carmichael. TEXT

They Called It Love, But Was It Love? Charan Singh. VIDEO

This Is Right; Zak, Life and After. Gevi Dimitrakopoulou. VIDEO

A Time to Listen. New York City AIDS Memorial. PROJECT

To Make the Wounded Whole: African American Responses to HIV/AIDS. Dan Royels. BOOK

We Both Laughed in Pleasure: The Selected Diaries of Lou Sullivan. Ellis Martin and Zach Ozma, eds. BOOK

"We Need a Plan for How to Have Casual Sex Again." Mathew Rodriguez. TEXT

"What Does a COVID-19 Doula Do?" What Would an HIV Doula Do? TEXT

2021

AIDS IS / AIDS AIN'T 40 Resource List. What Would an HIV Doula Do? PROJECT

AIDS, Posters, and Stories of Public Health: A People's History of a Pandemic. Theodore (ted) Kerr. EXHIBITION

Between Certain Death and a Possible Future: Queer Writing on Growing up with the AIDS Crisis. Mattilda Bernstein Sycamore, ed. BOOK

Detransition, Baby. Torrey Peters. BOOK

Forget Burial: HIV Kinship, Disability, and Queer/Trans Narratives of Care. Marty Fink. BOOK

Gay Bar: Why We Went Out. Jeremy Atherton Lin. BOOK

Gregg Bordowitz: I I Wanna Be Well. Peter Eleey. EXHIBITION

I Am . . . a Long-Term AIDS Survivor. Steed Taylor. VIDEO

I'm a Challenger: A Living Women's History of HIV/AIDS in the United States: Brooklyn, History Moves + STAR Program. BOOK + PROJECT

In the Future. Beto Pérez. VIDEO

It's a Sin. Russell T. Davies. VIDEO

Last Call: A True Story of Love, Lust, and Murder in Queer New York. Elon Green. BOOK

Let the Record Show: A Political History of ACT UP New York, 1987–1993. Sarah Schulman. BOOK

Love Your Asian Body: AIDS Activism in Los Angeles. Eric Wat. BOOK

#Medstrike: Confronting the Non-Profit Industrial Complex. Abdul-Aliy A. Muhammad w/ Uriah Bussey, #Medstrike: Confronting the Non-Profit Industrial Complex. VIDEO

The Mersey Model. Danny Kilbride. VIDEO

More Life. Robert Goff, Director Thor Shannon, and Associate Director Alec Smyth. EXHIBITION

Niki de Saint Phalle: Structures for Life. Ruba Katrib and Josephine Graf. EXHIBITION

100 Boyfriends. Brontez Purnell. BOOK

Palma Tilteá. Cristóbal Guerra. VIDEO

To End a Plague: America's Fight to Defeat AIDS in Africa. Emily Bass. BOOK

Voices at the Gate. Katherine Cheairs. VIDEO

Up against the Wall: Art, Activism, and the AIDS Poster. Donald Albrecht and Jessica Lacher-Feldman. BOOK.

The Viral Underclass: How Racism, Ableism and Capitalism Plague Humans on the Margins. Steven Thrasher. BOOK

The Women's Video Support Project. J Triangular. VIDEO

NOTES

INTRODUCTION

1 The Combahee River Collective Statement, Combahee River Collective, 1977, https://www.blackpast.org/african-american-history/combahee-river -collective-statement-1977/.

2 "When ACT UP Is Remembered, Other Places, People, and Forms of AIDS Activism Are Disremembered: Part Two of an Interview with Queer Archive Activist Alexandra Juhasz," Visual AIDS (blog), February 17, 2013, https://www .thebody.com/article/when-act-up-is-remembered-other-places-people-and-; "I Made My Mourning Productive, Collective, and Interactive through Video production . . ." Visual AIDS (blog), February 5, 2013, https://visualaids.org/blog /i-made-my-mourning-productive-collective-and-interactive-through-video -prod.

3 Jennifer Brier, *Infectious Ideas: US Political Responses to the AIDS Crisis* (Chapel Hill: University of North Carolina Press, 2009).

4 Ted Kerr, ed., "Time Is Not a Line," special issue, *We Who Feel Differently* 3 (Fall 2014), https://wewhofeeldifferently.info/journal.php.

5 Katherine McKittrick, *Dear Science and Other Stories* (Durham, NC: Duke University Press, 2021), 28.

6 "Metanoia: Transformation through AIDS Archives and Activism," ONE Archives Foundation, accessed November 14, 2021, https://www.onearchives.org /metanoia/.

7 Thanks to an anonymous reader for Duke University Press for these terms.

8 McKittrick, *Dear Science*, 31.

TRIGGER 1. WHAT WE SEE

1 Hito Steyerl, "In Defense of the Poor Image," *e-flux* 10 (November 2009), https://www.e-flux.com/journal/10/61362/in-defense-of-the-poor-image; Alexandra Juhasz, *Learning from YouTube* (Cambridge, MA: MIT Press, 2011), http:// vectors.usc.edu/projects/learningfromyoutube.

TRIGGER 2. SEEING TAPE IN TIME

1 For example, see Chris Collins, Tim Sweeney, John Boring, Michael Callen, and Keith Lawrence, "Who Knows What about Us?," *New York Native*, June 20, 1983.

2 To learn more about Whitbread and her practice, visit her website at http:// jessicawhitbread.com.

3 You can read the Denver Principles at OnCurating, no. 42 (2019), http://www .on-curating.org/issue-42-reader/the-denver-principles.html.

4 DIVA TV (Damned Interfering Video Activists), formed in 1989, were an important affinity group in ACT UP. See "DIVA TV," ACT UP NY, https://actupny .org/divatv.1.html. The Testing the Limits Collective formed in 1986 (David Meieran, Gregg Bordowitz, Robin Hutt, Sandra Elgear, and Jean Carlomusto) was constituted by graduates of the Independent Study Program of The Whitney Museum of American Art , which also added to the AIDS media activist scene artists like Ray Navarro, Catherine Gund, Ellen Spiro, and Tom Kalin. See Alexandra Juhasz, "'So Many Alternatives': The Alternative AIDS Video Movement," Cineaste 20, no. 4 (1994), https://actupny.org/diva/cineaste2.html #anchor930682.

5 Cathy J. Cohen, The Boundaries of Blackness: AIDS and the Breakdown of Black Politics (Chicago: University of Chicago Press, 1999).

6 Ellen Spiro, "What to Wear on Your Video Activist Outing (Because the Whole World Is Watching)," The Independent, May 1991.

7 Alexandra Juhasz, AIDS TV: Identity, Community, and Alternative Video (Durham, NC: Duke University Press, 1995).

8 John Greyson, "Strategic Compromises: AIDS and Alternative Video Practices," in Re-Imaging America: The Arts of Social Change, ed. Mark O'Brien and Craig Little (Philadelphia: New Society, 1990), 60–74.

9 Timothy Landers, "Bodies and Anti-Bodies: A Crisis in Representation," Independent 11, no. 1 (January/February 1988): 18–24.

10 Read about Rashidah Abdul-Khabeer in her own words in her oral history with Dan Royles for his African American AIDS Activism Oral History Project, http://afamaidshist.fiu.edu/omeka-s/s/african-american-aids-history-project /item/2549.

11 Dan Royles, To Make the Wounded Whole: The African American Struggle against HIV/AIDS (Chapel Hill: University of North Carolina Press, 2020).

12 Royles, To Make the Wounded Whole, 37.

13 Cindy Patton, "Heterosexual AIDS Panic: A Queer Paradigm," Gay Community News 12, no. 29 (February 9, 1985): 5–6.

14 Cohen, Boundaries of Blackness, ix.

TRIGGER 3. BEING TRIGGERED TOGETHER

1 VHS Archives, Center for Humanites, https://www.centerforthehumanities .org/public-engagement/working-groups/vhs-archives.

2 Jesse Cohen, Catherine Czacki, Taraneh Fazeli, Citron Kelly, Carolyn Lazard, Bonnie Swencionis, and Rebecca Watson Horn, "Canaries: Refuge in the Means," Recess, 2016, https://www.recessart.org/canaries/.

TRIGGER 4. BEING TRIGGERED IN TIMES

1　Ray Navarro and Catherine Saalfied [Gund], "Seeing through AIDS: Media Workshop Guide" (New York: Media Network, 1990).
2　See Catherine Saalfield [Gund], "Videography," in *AIDS TV: Identity, Community, and Alternative Video* (Durham, NC: Duke University Press, 1995), 271–76.
3　Dan Royles, *To Make the Wounded Whole: The African American Struggle against HIV/AIDS* (Chapel Hill: University of North Caroling Press, 2020), 41.
4　Karl McCool, personal comments during "(re)Presenting AIDS: Culture and Accountability," Visual AIDS, CUNY Grad Center, 2013.
5　Stefano Harney, Fred Moten, and Stevphen Shukaitis, "Studying through the Undercommons," Class War University, November 12, 2012, https://classwaru.org /2012/11/12/studying-through-the-undercommons-stefano-harney-fred-moten -interviewed-by-stevphen-shukaitis/.

TRIGGER 5. BEING TRIGGERED BY ABSENCE

1　Tina Campt, *Listening to Images* (Durham, NC: Duke University Press, 2017).
2　Campt, "Introduction: Listening to Images: An Exercise in Counterintuition," in *Listening to Images*, 3–11.

TRIGGER 6. HOW TO HAVE
AN AIDS MEMORIAL IN AN EPIDEMIC

1　See VOCAL's website for more information: http://www.vocal-ny.org.
2　Paul Sendziuk, Roger Hallas, Jim Hubbard, and Debra Levine, "Moving Pictures: AIDS on Film and Video," *GLQ* 16, no. 3 (2010), 429–49.
3　To learn more about the history of ACT UP political funerals, visit ACT UP NY: https://actupny.org/diva/polfunsyn.html.
4　Douglas Crimp, "Mourning and Militancy," *October* 51 (Winter 1989): 3–18.
5　James Young, *The Stages of Memory: Reflections on Memorial Art, Loss, and the Spaces Between* (Public History in Historical Perspective) (Amherst: University of Massachusetts Press, 2016).
6　Alexandra Juhasz, "Digital AIDS Documentary: Webs, Rooms, Viruses, and Quilts," in *Blackwell Companion to Documentary*, ed. Alexandra Juhasz and Alisa Lebow (Cambridge, MA: Blackwell, 2015), 314–34.
7　Emilie Townes, *Womanist Ethics and the Cultural Production of Evil* (London: Palgrave Macmillan, 2006), 22.
8　Dagmawi Woubshet, *The Calendar of Loss: Race, Sexuality, and Mourning in the Early Era of AIDS* (Baltimore: Johns Hopkins University Press, 2015).
9　Alex Fialho's description of his tribute walks is available at Visual AIDS, accessed November 14, 2021, https://visualaids.org/blog/alex-fialho-writes -about-his-last-address-tribute-walk.

253

NOTES

7. SILENCE + OBJECT

1 VHS Archives, Center for the Humanities, https://www.centerforthehumanities
   .org/public-engagement/working-groups/vhs-archives.
2 Gabriele Griffin, *Visibility Blue/s: Representations of HIV and AIDS* (Manchester,
   UK: Manchester University Press, 2000).
3 Douglas Crimp, "Mourning and Militancy," *October* 51 (Winter 1989): 3–18.

8. SILENCE + ART

1 Learn more about My Barbarian at https://mybarbarian.com/About.
2 "Social Determinants of Health," World Health Organization, accessed November 14, 2021, https://www.who.int/social_determinants/en/.
3 Ryan Conrad, ed., *Against Equality: Queer Revolution, Not Mere Inclusion* (Chico,
   CA: AK, 2014).

9. SILENCE + VIDEO

1 See "Global Forum on MSM and HIV," https://www.unaids.org/en/resources
   /multimediacentre/photos/2008/20080802globalforumonmsmandhiv.
2 "When ACT UP Is Remembered, Other Places, People, and Forms of AIDS
   Activism Are Disremembered: Part Two of an Interview with Queer Archive
   Activist Alexandra Juhasz," *Visual AIDS* (blog), February 17, 2013, https://www
   .thebody.com/article/when-act-up-is-remembered-other-places-people-and-;
   "I Made My Mourning Productive, Collective, and Interactive through Video
   production..." *Visual AIDS* (blog), February 5, 2013, https://visualaids.org/blog
   /i-made-my-mourning-productive-collective-and-interactive-through-video
   -prod.
3 Smithsonian Institution, Archives of American Art, Visual Arts and the AIDS
   Epidemic: An Oral History Project, "Oral History Interview with Alexandra
   Juhasz, 2017 December 19–21," https://www.aaa.si.edu/collections/interviews
   /oral-history-interview-alexandra-juhasz-17531.
4 "*Exhibition: One on One Project*. Photography by Ted Kerr, Curatorial Statement
   by Q. C. Gu," *Prairie Artsters* (blog),December 14, 2009, http://prairieartsters
   .blogspot.com/2009/12/exhibition-one-on-one-project.html.

10. SILENCE + UNDETECTABILITY

1 Learn more about the history of U = U at Prevention Access, https://www
   .preventionaccess.org/about.
2 See the project at "The Undetectables," https://liveundetectable.org/.
3 Personal communication, LGBT Center, New York, April 29, 2019

11. SILENCE + CONVERSATION

1   David Oscar Harvey, Marty Fink, Alexandra Juhasz, and Bishnu Gosh, "Ghost Stories," *Jump Cut* 55 (Fall 2013), https://www.ejumpcut.org/archive/jc55.2013/AidsHivIntroduction/index.html.

2   Hugh Ryan, "How to Whitewash a Plague," *New York Times*, August 3, 2013.

3   Hugh Ryan, "(re)Presenting AIDS: Culture and Accountability," Visual AIDS, August 20, 2013, https://visualaids.org/events/detail/representing-aids-culture-and-accountability.

4   Ryan, "(re)Presenting AIDS."

5   Alexandra Juhasz, "Forgetting ACT UP," *Quarterly Journal of Speech* 98, no. 1 (2012): 69–74.

6   "What You Don't Know Could Fill a Museum: AIDS, Art and the Institution," Visual AIDS, January 4, 2014, https://www.visualaids.org/events/detail/what-you-dont-know-could-fill-a-museum-activism-aids-art-and-the-institutio.

7   "As We Canonize Certain Producers of Culture We Are Closing Space for a Complication of Narratives," Visual AIDS, December 10, 2013, https://visualaids.org/blog/as-we-canonize-certain-producers-of-culture-we-are-closing-space-for-a-comp.

8   Lucas Hilderbrand, "Retroactivism," *GLQ* 12, no. 2 (April 2006): 303–17.

12. SILENCE + INTERACTION

1   Mark King, My Fabulous Disease (blog), accessed November 14, 2021, https://marksking.com/.

2   Dion Kagan, *Positive Images: Gay Men and HIV/AIDS in the Culture of "Post Crisis"* (London: I. B. Tauris, 2018).

3   Adam M. Geary, *Antiblack Racism and the AIDS Epidemic* (London: Palgrave Macmillan, 2014).

4   Theodore Kerr, "AIDS 1969: HIV, History, and Race," *Drain Magazine* 13, no. 2 (2016), http://drainmag.com/aids-1969-hiv-history-and-race/; Robert F. Garry, "Documentation of an AIDS Virus Infection in the United States in 1968," *JAMA* 260, no. 14 (November 1988): 2085–87; Randy Shilts, *And the Band Played On* (New York: St. Martin's Press, 1987).

5   Personal communication, New York, January 2015.

6   Jih-Fei Cheng, "AIDS, Black Feminisms, and the Institutionalization of Queer Politics," *GLQ* 25, no. 1 (January 2019): 169–77.

7   You can read the Tacoma Action Collective #StopErasingBlackPeople press release at OnCurating, no. 42 (2019), http://www.on-curating.org/issue-42-reader/stoperasingblackpeople.html#.XboWLmRKhhA.

8   Read more at "Bottom-Up History: An Interview with StoryCorps' Dave Isay," The Millions, January 13, 2011, https://themillions.com/2011/01/bottom-up-history-an-interview-with-storycorps-dave-isay.html.

9   See Stephen Vider, https://www.stephenvider.com/queerness-of-home.

10 Learn more about the exhibition at Visual AIDS, "Everyday," November 17–
December 10, 2016, https://visualaids.org/events/detail/everyday.

13. SILENCE + TRANSFORMATION

1 Learn more about the collective at HIV Doula Work, http://hivdoula.work/.
2 "Past Present Future: The Ongoing AIDS Epidemic in Four Documents,"
Union Docs, January 11, 2018, https://uniondocs.org/event/2018-01-11-past
-present-future.
3 ACT UP Women's Committee, *Women AIDS and Activism* (Boston: South End,
1992).

CONCLUSION

1 In the process of writing this conclusion, we explored many cultural moments
and objects that challenged and stretched our thinking, including the TV show
Pose, Donald Trump's 2017 State of the Union Address, the play *A Strange Loop*
by Michael Jackson, and the exhibition *On Our Backs* at Leslie-Lohman Museum in New York, curated by Alexis Heller. We wrote about Normalization
through the lens of *On Our Backs* for *X-tra*. Our thinking about Normalization
has changed since that writing.
2 We have both contributed widely to this discourse. To see some of our work
and that of others, visit the resource we created as part of the 27 Questions
Project and a set of COVID-19 specific zines with What Would an HIV Doula
Do? Collective at HIV Doula Work, http://hivdoula.work/27-questions (accessed November 14, 2021).

SOURCES AND INFLUENCES

1 TL Cowan, "Citation Is Not Enough," https://scalar.usc.edu/nehvectors
/100hardtruths-fakenews/93-citation-is-not-enough.

INDEX

Abdul-Khabeer, Rashidah, 32–40, 63–64, 80–81

Abramson, Mark, 161

Acquavella, Demien, 218–19. See also *Can You Bring It? Bill T. Jones and D-Man in the Water*

"A.D. 2000," 87. *See also* Erykah Badu

Adesegun, Nathylin Flowers, 210–12

AIDS/HIV: activism, 1, 3, 31–38, 42, 59–60, 75, 85, 107, 148, 161, 170, 175, 190; activists videos, 1, 8, 29, 32–36, 39, 44, 54, 68–69, 75, 158, 190, 236; and Black women, 8–9, 36, 43, 81–84, 180, 199, 201, 204, 213; and dance, 44, 148, 161, 217–19, 222–25; epidemic, 2–3, 12, 43, 78, 81, 83, 85–88, 91, 110, 119, 134–40, 176, 186, 220–24; and First Nations, 130, 190; and gay white men, 12, 32, 36, 148, 161, 186, 199, 209; and the internet, 37, 55–56, 67, 69, 114, 144, 179; media ecology of, 39, 42, 45, 85; memorials, 1, 87–91, 106, 225; protests, 1, 55, 170–72, 223; responses to, 36, 46, 68, 81, 89, 102–4, 114–15, 119, 125–29, 135–37, 140, 156–61, 179, 194, 199, 202–3, 209, 213; and sex workers, 11, 35; statistics, 13; and undetectability, 162–68; and women, 3, 8, 11, 25–37, 41–46, 55, 63–68, 71, 75, 79–80, 107, 129, 149–50, 153, 172, 176, 181, 186, 190, 195–201, 205–6, 212, 228. *See also* AIDS Crisis Culture; AIDS [Crisis] Normalization; AIDS Crisis Revisitation; Bebashi; Black women; First Silence; Second Silence; silence; Times of AIDS; trigger

AIDS at Home, 194. *See also* Vider, Stephen

AIDS Before AIDS, 218

An AIDS Conversation Script to be Read Aloud: Timeline, 2, 6, 10, 95

AIDS Crisis Culture, xiii, 6–7, 9, 11, 35, 39, 47, 55, 62, 64, 68, 75, 79, 88, 96, 101, 106–15, 118, 127, 136, 140, 147, 149, 159, 164, 175–78, 183; and dance 217–19, 222–25.

AIDS [Crisis] Normalization, xiv, 1, 7, 96–97, 219–22; and COVID-19, 223–24

AIDS Crisis Revisitation, xiv, 6–7, 10–12, 89, 96, 101–7, 113, 155, 159–88, 191, 194, 198, 203, 206, 209, 213–14, 219, 222–25.

AIDS Cultural Production, 1–11, 13, 30–31, 35, 38–39, 42, 47, 57, 78, 85, 90–91, 103, 108, 113–15, 127–29, 159, 175–77, 181–84, 192, 220, 223, 227

AIDS in NYC: The First Five Years, 172, 175

AIDS TV, 54, 59, 109

Anderson, Wesley, 41

And the Band Played On (1987), 188

anti-Black racism, 2, 183, 187

Art AIDS America, 191, 194

Ashe, Arthur, 36

Ayotte, Zachary, 137

Badu, Erykah, 87, 92

Basinger, Joanne, 45

Bebashi: Transition to Hope, 7–10, 27, 40–42, 46, 49–50, 52, 63, 65, 70, 73–74, 78–81, 84–92, 103, 186, 204, 206, 218; videotape, 7, 9, 19–24, 29, 30–37, 43, 52, 70, 73, 78, 81, 84, 101, 106. *See also* Black women; "Grandma's Legacy"

Bell, Gary J., 81

Bennett, Miriam, 26–27. See also "Grandma's Legacy"

Bennett, Ms., 26–28, 44–45, 87. *See also* "Grandma's Legacy"

Berkowitz, Richard, 32, 171–72

Biggest Quake, The, 161

258

INDEX